I TATTI STUDIES IN
ITALIAN RENAISSANCE HISTORY

Sponsored by Villa I Tatti
Harvard University Center for Italian Renaissance Studies
Florence, Italy

EVERYDAY RENAISSANCES

The Quest for Cultural Legitimacy in Venice

SARAH GWYNETH ROSS

Harvard University Press

Cambridge, Massachusetts

London, England

2016

Printed in the United States of America

First printing

Library of Congress Cataloging-in-Publication Data

Ross, Sarah Gwyneth, 1975-
Everyday Renaissances : the quest for cultural legitimacy in Venice / Sarah Gwyneth Ross.
pages cm
Includes bibliographical references and index.
ISBN 978-0-674-65983-4 (alk. paper)
1. Renaissance—Italy—Venice. 2. Philosophy, Renaissance. 3. Physicians—Italy—Venice—History—16th century. 4. Middle class—Italy—Venice—History—16th century. 5. Middle class—Italy—Venice—History—17th century. 6. Venice (Italy)—Civilization—To 1797. 7. Venice (Italy)—Intellectual life—16th century. I. Title.
CB361.R67 2016
940.2′1—dc23

2015030883

In ammirazione di Francesco Longo,
filosofo, dovunque sia

CONTENTS

EVERYDAY RENAISSANCES

INTRODUCTION

This book is about the Renaissance, but not the era's literary or artistic celebrities. Our subjects are Venetian men and women living outside the circles of power and the Renaissances they experienced and represented. We will be examining a world of aspiration inhabited by people who valued learning and literature but whose families lacked formal political authority and whose intellectual lives were not coterminous with their gainful employment. Patronage networks were not ready-made for them, and cachet did not form part of their patrimony. For the subjects of this book, moreover, education was often a gift, not a given. Learning provided our protagonists with the tools to interpret and improve their lives, to make the world around them; their different forms of contact with books and learning elevated, transformed, or anchored them, depending on their points of origin, where they aimed to go, and what hopes they cherished for kin, colleagues, and friends in future generations.

Scholars and broader audiences alike now tend to level charges of elitism at "the Renaissance" as a cultural phenomenon, and with some justice. Patrons of culture had uncommon wealth. And even if most producers of culture had relatively humble origins, they enjoyed uncommon talent. Yet *Everyday Renaissances* claims that ordinary people also participated energetically in culture, and that attending to them offers a sharper picture of the era's intellectual and literary ferment. I do not, however, aim to revive Jacob Burckhardt's conception of egalitarianism in Renaissance Italy.[1] Our protagonists seldom reveal a utopia of cultural accessibility; more often they tell us of their effort to possess books, education, and literary esteem.

Even their successes—and there were successes—reveal the social tensions they confronted.

Looking at the cultural and intellectual lives of predominantly unheralded artisanal, mercantile, and professional people with little discretionary income or leisure, we confront an essential question: What did culture do for people? The scholarship of the last half century has taught us that literary, intellectual, or artistic work and its sponsorship always had practical dimensions. If it requires little argument that Leonardo da Vinci needed to eat, we have had to think carefully about the complex ways in which literary and artistic patronage supported the careers of scholars and artists while at the same time enhancing the reputations and serving the objectives of their patrons.[2] When we move into society's middle ranks, questions of culture's value and its practical applications become both more pressing and more difficult to answer. Could the allocation of resources to literary or artistic studies repay the effort in the cases of people for whom prominent roles in the republic of letters, the academies, or even the civil professions would be unlikely?[3] This study answers that question in the affirmative, although focusing on books and education far more than visual art. The Renaissance mattered to everyday people, because even provisional contact with intellectual and literary endeavors built reputations, initiated or continued processes of social mobility, and promised an honorable posterity.

Resting on an evidentiary base of more than four thousand archival documents, especially wills, household inventories, and account books, this study showcases diverse fragments of cultural experience. Making sense of those fragments and their owners, however, requires a new theoretical framework. I would like to begin, then, by highlighting a representative artifact and drawing out the framework in which it can be situated before surveying this book's sources, protagonists, and specific interventions.

ONE RETAILER, TWO GREEK MANUSCRIPTS, AND A THEORY OF CULTURAL LEGITIMACY

On June 18, 1556, a Venetian secondhand goods dealer named Francesco entrusted his shop boy, Zuanne, with an interesting errand. Zuanne was to procure two Greek manuscripts from His Magnificence, Andrea di Franceschi, a secretary of the ducal chancery whose duties included granting permission to borrow items from the collection of books and manuscripts that would, centuries later, still form the core of Venice's famous library, the Biblioteca Nazionale di San Marco. The ledgers that Franceschi kept most often reveal the usual suspects of libraries: career scholars, orators, secretaries, writers, and lawyers. But a few physicians also appeared and even, on this occasion, a minor player in the world of commerce. His Magnificence may have been taken aback to find a retail merchant attempting to make use of the lending potential of this collection, but in any event he took the basin that Zuanne had brought as surety and made this note: "18 June 1556, Mr. Francesco (son of Paul), who runs a second-hand shop near the clock tower in the Piazza San Marco, has borrowed a Greek book on parchment called *Proclus on Platonic Theology* and also *The Commentary of Hierocles on the Golden Verses of Pythagoras,* which his servant, Zuanne of Venice, will take to him with my permission. And I have had from him as a collateral an engraved silver basin."[4] The desire of a secondhand goods dealer to borrow two Greek manuscripts treating philosophy encapsulates the point of this study: literary culture mattered, for a host of reasons, to everyday people in Renaissance Europe. More specifically, I am arguing that literature mattered to Venetian men and women who, like this retailer, did not belong to the political or even cultural elite. Some left discursive evidence of how the humanities enriched their minds and souls; however, they more often reveal how contact with the literary helped them earn respect (including self-respect), cover social blemishes, and, in some cases, improve their social positions. Cultural legitimacy as a concept makes room for both inherent value and its potential instrumental applications.[5]

Why, more particularly, might a secondhand goods dealer such as messer Francesco have wanted to consult Greek manuscripts? Like many of the sources at the heart of this book, these lending records are laconic, making the task of divining motives even more problematic than usual. But any purely practical motive we might give him would lead us to unlikelihood. If he had come into possession of similar manuscripts and wanted to verify their authenticity or completeness as part of assessing their value, it would have been more efficient to enlist the services of a humanist or grammarian. Might messer Francesco himself have possessed sufficient knowledge of Greek and philosophy? A secondhand goods dealer could have been the well-educated son of a patrician or citizen family that suffered economic decline. By the middle of the sixteenth century, many families in Venice responded to financial constriction by practicing extreme estate planning, effectively disinheriting most children to transmit the estate intact to the most capable heir. Such a strategy required monachating many daughters and sons, as well as pushing other boys either into commercial apprenticeships, or else providing the minimal support for university studies that might prepare the young men for a learned profession.[6] Francesco might have had such a story, and in that case perhaps the requisite skills to read and comprehend the manuscripts unaided. But we would still have to ask why he did not interact with this material in printed form. Proclus, for instance, was widely available, and in 1516 had even appeared in a scholarly Aldine edition. Why go to the trouble of sending an employee to fetch these manuscripts, which required making collateral of a precious object, as well as time and inconvenience? Attempting to give this man a practical aim leads us to rationales such as an aversion to print media or a second career as a humanist that would be highly improbable (though admittedly not impossible) for a man described as a retailer.

We thus have an instance of bibliophilia that requires a different category of analysis than the ones intellectual historians tend to use. While we cannot be certain of Francesco's specific motive, it fell between the quasi-professional exigencies animating people deeply embedded in and identified with the world of literature and the vagaries of aspiration, curiosity, practical need, and pleasure pushing amateurs toward literary material. We need a framework for understanding cases such as this that fall between our usual interpretive categories, but one that does not establish a mutual exclusivity between the typologies at either end. "Cultural legitimacy" allows for appreciating degrees of difference—comparatively grand or comparatively modest educational or expressive ambition, a monumental or a modest collection of books, a tight or a tenuous connection to an intellectual community—while still keeping an overarching set of shared values in view. We can appreciate the differences between a celebrated humanist such as Pietro Bembo and a goldsmith's wife who harbored an Italian rendering of Ovid's *Metamorphoses,* yet still see how both historical actors occupied a field of endeavor that their era charged with social no less than literary meanings.

Returning to those manuscripts at San Marco, one thing is clear: Everyone who appeared in these lending records, whether literary celebrities or retailers, had easier access to the same material by other routes. These volumes, the most famous texts of pagan antiquity and medieval theology, had printed editions easily accessible in Venice. This city, still the print capital of Europe, housed hundreds of printers who collectively produced between fifteen thousand and thirty thousand volumes annually.[7] Elite borrowers with general interests and anyone connected to them, moreover, also would already have enjoyed access to manuscript versions through friendship networks. The only major category of borrowers, then, who could have needed these manuscripts were humanists, who might require a particular redaction for their research. Borrowers who were not humanists by definition, and perhaps even those who were, must then have derived as much benefit from participating in the community that formed around this collection as they did from the volumes themselves. Even the most recondite exchanges of literati were, as Christopher Celenza observes, "as much social and involved with the search for distinction" as they were scholarly.[8] In the case of the Marciana collection, by borrowing a manuscript the individual formed or strengthened an ennobling connection to the literary life of their city. Francesco the secondhand goods dealer might have had a fascinating background and myriad pursuits, but he was described as a secondhand goods dealer. Yet in the act of borrowing these two Greek manuscripts he inscribed himself in a small way as part of the same Renaissance culture inhabited by luminaries like Giovanni Battista Ramusio, a heavy borrower in these years.[9] In other words, messer Francesco obtained a measure of honor connected to educational and literary attainment that had the power to reshape his self-perception, reputation, and potentially even his or his children's social position. That type of honor is what I am calling *cultural legitimacy*.

But cultural legitimacy needs a more precise definition. It will be best to begin with what this concept is not—or, more accurately, what it is not quite or not only. Cultural legitimacy relates to but is not quite meritocracy. Like meritocracy, cultural legitimacy indicates the prioritization of earned distinctions and skills over inherited status or material assets. But meritocracy, in its literal definition if not in common usage, denotes the conferral specifically of political power on the basis of proven abilities, rather than birth or wealth. Meritocracy's loose and depoliticized modern connotation would be close to what I mean by cultural legitimacy, but its denotation goes wide of the mark. Indeed, the term *legitimacy* itself often connects to legally constituted governmental authority (or claims thereto), but with the modifier *cultural* I mean to indicate a fundamental distinction between this political usage and my own meaning. This book treats matters of the mind, not the mechanisms or representations of governance.

Closer to my interests is the sociologist Pierre Bourdieu's notion of "cultural capital," which I will indeed apply in certain instances.[10] Yet as much as I share Bourdieu's conviction that abstract merits have tangible value, his concept privileges too much the ultimate conversion of intellectual, literary, and artistic possessions and commitments into literal social and economic rewards.[11] Cultural legitimacy embraces the potential of that socioeconomic conversion; indeed, we will see several individuals leveraging their intellectual honor to dignify their professions, broker prestigious marriages for their children, and initiate (or continue) processes of generational social mobility within their families. But cultural legitimacy, at least in the early-modern Venetian context, was not only about practical gain and social positioning. Intellectual and literary values had a power that was not always measurable, let alone monetary. If meritocracy had too much of the political, cultural capital has too much of the economic to be fully satisfactory here.[12]

If these are the interpretive structures whose limitations urge analytical renovation, the work of art historians and scholars of material culture, above all Renata Ago, have inspired the major design features of the category I am proposing. Ago in particular draws from household inventories of seventeenth-century Rome a fascinating survey of the art, luxury goods, musical instruments, and books collected by an impressive swath of society, from artisans to patricians.[13] Beyond finding ordinary collectors worlds away from an Isabella d'Este, she expresses eloquently the social meanings ascribed to the interactions between object and owner. Lorna Weatherill has used this line of reasoning to compelling effect in her analysis of English consumption of books, art, and other "luxury" goods at the end of the early-modern period.[14] But Ago has gone the furthest in theorizing the meanings of those interactions, which, she claims, signaled individuals' "quasi-noble lifestyle," or an ostensibly impractical "taste" that marked them as cultivated.[15] Even book owners with only a few volumes beyond devotional material, she suggests, proved that they were "intellectuals of a modest sort."[16]

Ago makes space for forms of social motion impossible in Bourdieu's model. Within what he called the "aristocracy of culture" intellectuals of a modest sort suffered exclusion. While he envisioned provisional possibilities for individuals to move in and out of the cultural aristocracy, he understood social boundaries as vigilantly policed and sites of a "permanent struggle."[17] One might join this aristocracy, but only by internalizing and reproducing its *habitus*—styles of education, comportment, possession, and display, but above all modes of thought and perception—to the point that it became owned, automatic, habitual.[18] Those lacking complete knowledge or impeccable credentials, such as autodidacts (whether partial or complete) or anyone without a university degree, he insisted, suffer either relegation to the margins or exclusion from "the legitimate culture."[19] The rigidity of Bourdieu's formulation even encompasses the claim that working-class men and women actively participate in their exclusion by putting moral boundaries between their hardworking virtue and the perceived corruption of elites. Those falling between the ranks of cultural aristocrats and the working classes, in his system, can be positive members only of the petit bourgeoisie itself, and in reality only certain sectors even within that already restricted group. Minute shadings of status connected to family, education and income define sub-ranks. In Bourdieu's model, then, the person of modest intellectual or other cultural attainments necessarily faces the hostility of the culturally rich and culturally poor alike.

By contrast, Ago emphasizes the interstices of early-modern social hierarchies, where she locates an "elite of taste, defined by the possession of cultural goods whose value had to do with their beauty, ingenuity or innovativeness more than the cost of their materials. Lacking any other sort of visible distinction or testimonial, whether direct or indirect, their cultural material vouched for them."[20] Less tethered than Bourdieu to hermeneutics of class conflict and market economics, but still attentive to the problem of social boundaries and culture's role in reproducing them, Ago's "elite of taste" captures better the dynamics of premodern Europe.

But who formed Ago's more flexible elite? "Amid the middle ranks of the population," she explains, lay "a group that wanted to be appreciated as 'cultivated,' 'trendy,' 'refined,' and who invested their respectability in those traits," rather than wealth, station, or office as such.[21] Ago and I study the same types of people, and I find evocative the range of terms she has devised for expressing their hopes—and even more so the ways those terms interact. She speaks variously of taste, cultivation, trendiness, and refinement. Yet it is never quite clear to whom this elite of taste displayed their cultural credentials. That audience could not be the socioeconomic elite, as some members of that group (lawyers, for instance, or minor patricians) also belonged to the elite of taste. Nor, beyond a general desire for respectability, does Ago suggest the goals that motivated her protagonists or tell us whether or not those goals were fulfilled. Admittedly, the fluidity of Ago's model is part of what makes it so attractive. But a scholar who is at least in part a social historian wants more stable rubrics. Cultivation and trendiness can interact but are manifestly not the same thing. And even cultivation and refinement need not be coterminous. Combined and juxtaposed, then, these different qualities ably describe Ago's subjects; however, she offers no unified theory for them, nor can any of these terms stand on its own as a heuristic tool. Cultivation comes close, but we must ask cultivated in what particular sense, to what specific end(s), and in dialogue with whom? Ago offers provocative case studies of individuals, but how did they interact with each other, if not literally, at least in their values and practices?

The category of legitimacy I am offering brings us back to the relational, but it allows for a positive inclusiveness of the sort Ago imagined and Bourdieu denied. Access to the literary created possibilities for joining a cultural lineage, but one not restricted by bloodlines or formal networks.[22] At the same time, cultural legitimacy examined within the particular realm of literary priorities refines Ago's more general notion of the quest for "respectability," positing a specific realm of endeavor in which self-defined "people of taste" interacted and the norms that helped define their interactions. The norms I have in mind include the veneration of antiquity or of the modern authors who revered and imitated antiquity, a confidence in the polyvalent value of education, and an emphasis on academic or literary credentials in the process of constructing individual, professional, or family honor. These priorities set general parameters for making claims to cultural legitimacy but did not constitute a rigid *habitus*.

This emphasis on relationship also keeps us more attuned to early-modern modes of thought. As economic and social historians alike have taught us, the early-modern world ran on systems of credit, in all senses of the word, which were defined not by mathematical formulae, let alone sociological models. Instead, early-modern men and women earned credit from the reputations they forged in sometimes rapidly changing sociopolitical environments and within unpredictable networks of human relationship.[23] In thinking about legitimacy, we also get a useful stimulus to ponder different levels and forms of belonging. Indeed, belonging gives the term *legitimacy* its greatest analytical power. Cultural legitimacy meant belonging to a lineage defined by commitment to intellectual, literary, or artistic matters. Commitment, not expertise or even necessarily competency, served as the minimum requirement for affiliation.

The value of belonging, however tenuously, to this lineage derived from the entrenchment of humanistic values. While humanists continued doing the precise philological, editorial, and authorial work that defined their particular neoclassical enterprise, the broader ideals that had inspired and justified that enterprise since its inception continued to take root in their social worlds. Those broader ideals included optimism about the ennobling power of education and a conception of the literary as an essential route to and proof of "virtue." By our period, humanists had spent two centuries propounding these more abstract notions as they packaged their program of study for diverse audiences. Society listened to those ideals, even while it did most of its reading in the vernacular—if at all.

Cultural legitimacy, then, indicates a continuum of relational humanistic values. By displaying an education if not always a deeply classical one, a literary inclination if not always a literary gift (let alone a publication record), the ownership of literature if not always a well-stocked library, the Renaissance subject showed that he or she belonged to one degree or another in the ranks of the cultured, the diverse "elite of taste" as Ago calls them, or people "of the right sort," as my Venetian protagonists usually express it. The degree of belonging might be close and tight, such as Ramusio's, or distant and loose, such as that, apparently, of Francesco the secondhand goods dealer. Cultural legitimacy can accommodate even tremendous differences of degree that were not ultimately differences of kind.

SOURCES AND PROTAGONISTS

Our protagonists are Venetian men and women living in the sixteenth and early seventeenth centuries. They are artisans, merchants, priests, lawyers, physicians, and their kin whom I have located in 3,005 Venetian testaments and 1,227 household inventories. These notarial records enable both wide-angle views of the city's cultural topography and detailed analysis of the literary lives of individuals who often left us nothing in libraries but sometimes a great deal in the archives. I also draw on manuscript *ricordanze,* as well as printed literature to explore different forms of access to, hopes for, and uses of cultural legitimacy. Out of these thousands of Venetians from the middle ranks of society, 147 men and women receive attention as book owners (101 souls) or practitioners of what I am terming *testamentary humanism* (46 souls). Within that group, approximately twenty individuals emerge with some detail, and three become central case studies: Nicolò Massa, Francesco Longo, and Alberto Rini.

These three core protagonists were all physicians, as were many of the others whose wills and household inventories reveal ardent devotion to the literary and eagerness for others to know about it. Physicians might not seem at first glance to be ideal guides to the literary lives of middling-sort Venetians. While historians generally conceive of physicians as enfranchised, in socioprofessional if not necessarily political or economic terms, a closer look at their circumstances as a group urges rethinking that conception.

Physicians became an unexpected focus of research and writing. This study grew out of a chance encounter with the uncharacteristically wordy, semiautobiographical testaments of Francesco Longo and questions about why a physician would seem so hungry for recognition as a man of wide experience and learning. Why did he not feel that as a physician he had sufficient honor or, in the terms I am suggesting, cultural legitimacy? Longo was even the son of an apothecary, but his university credentials (the requisite bachelor's degree the liberal arts and doctorate in medicine) brought considerable prestige. And his children might have continued his own story of social mobility; Longo's professional status paved the way for greater honor. Why, then, did he feel compelled to dictate two wills that drew not only on tropes of Christian piety but also on lessons in magnanimity derived from Plutarch—a fascinating case of humanistic special pleading?[24]

In the course of trying to understand this particular physician and his milieu, I formed larger questions about intellectual honor that his wills raised. Looking for others who exhibited similar preoccupations, I found many Venetians making ethical bequests in wills, possessing literary even if numerically small collections of books, and expressing concern for the intellectual formation of their children. Still, physicians consistently demonstrated themselves both most inclined to exploit the discursive potential of the testament and to harbor book collections that outpaced those of patricians by orders of magnitude, and even those of their near relatives on the professional family tree—priests, lawyers, secretaries—by significant margins.

Nancy Siraisi's pathbreaking work on the cross-pollination of historical and medical writing has taught us not to be surprised to find trained medical doctors doing literary work ostensibly unrelated to their primary careers.[25] But I also detected defensiveness, if not an anxiety, on that point. If Siraisi has demonstrated that physicians did a great deal of historical and antiquarian writing, it is worth questioning why—especially why practicing physicians seemed so desperate to draw attention to their broader literary pursuits, more than even their contributions to medical humanism as such.

The scholarship on humanism and the professions now generally posits that the long tradition of literary attacks on physicians as manual laborers with delusions of grandeur had subsided by the sixteenth century, when medicine had achieved a reasonably stable place, alongside the law, as a civil profession.[26] Yet on closer inspection, physicians protested, if not too much at least a good deal, about their humanistic learning and the need for society to give their profession more credit as a liberal art. These protests suggest medical doctors' fear that contemporaries still viewed their work as baser than that of the other learned professions, in part thanks to its unavoidable contact with human bodies. Medical doctors' repeated emphasis on these concerns indicates that medicine was still fighting for recognition as *scientia* not just *ars*. Contemporary dialogues, plays, and other forms of reception underscore the notion that the medicine remained suspect and, more than the other professions, relegated to a lesser order of endeavor than "pure" literary activity.

Both archival and print trails portray physicians and their families less as comfortable members of the urban elite and more as a group still in search of credibility. Put another way, when we examine the sources they did not intend for publication (and even some of those they did) physicians look less like privileged *cittadini* and more like harried occupants of the last rungs on the ladder of upward mobility. Indeed, in many cases physicians, like Longo, had artisanal or mercantile parentage. If the higher clergy, lawyers, ambassadors, and secretaries had put a safe distance between themselves and the taint of artisanal labor, physicians had not; they inhabited a tense space between those assumed to belong to the cultural elite and those who were assumed to be unlettered, or at least unliterary. Medical doctors labored under the peculiar tension of being "so close and yet so far" from the most secure forms of belonging on the spectrum of cultural legitimacy. Accordingly, I am arguing that while physicians' peculiar status made them more vocal than others about the cultural assets they hoped and trusted would distinguish them, they remained representative of the artisanal and mercantile worlds in that hope and trust. Patricians seldom worried about their intellectual or literary credentials; they had less to prove. Trying too hard, as Bourdieu pointed out long ago, is a sure sign of exclusion.[27]

In the positive sense, however, physicians' anxious rhetoric articulated a conviction in the ennobling and enriching potential of letters that those in the social ranks behind them also held but revealed in more laconic statements or gestured toward in their testamentary bequests of books or provisions for education. Physicians also reveal the various ways in which the idea of "enrichment" or "ennoblement" at the heart of cultural legitimacy might be conceived and used. Longo seems to have viewed that enrichment in a more personal sense; he worried less about his family's social mobility and more about crafting an image of himself as a learned man and bequeathing his essential philosophical precepts to his heirs. Many of his colleagues voiced their hopes of converting cultural legitimacy into social mobility. Some took pride in their family members' gradual integration with patricians—if not yet at the level of forming direct family ties, at least in terms of moving in patrician circles and enjoying greater latitude for dispensing patronage in their own right. A few physicians also became explicit defenders of the literary value of the medical profession.

Physicians thus lead us to particularly rich veins of evidence for anatomizing cultural legitimacy, but that evidence is by no means unique. Other categories of people within Venice's broad reading public shared physicians' central concerns. We will consider diverse stories of encounters with and hopes for books, education, and the next generation. If physicians could use the humanities as an astringent to sanitize a profession whose more distasteful responsibilities included smelling urine, other types of people found the humanities an effective cosmetic for covering their social blemishes, such as illegitimacy, or parents who were servants or artisans.

SCHOLARLY CONVERSATIONS

Beyond the analytical category it proposes and the variety of historical actors it recovers, *Everyday Renaissances* contributes methodologically to the growing rapprochement between intellectual and social history. Few of this book's protagonists have earned any notice from modern scholars, in part because they awaited recovery from the archival record. But people like this are also less apt to draw scholarly inquiry because they fall between two major sets of concerns. Intellectual historians still tend to focus on authors, or writers who left behind compositions intended for readers beyond themselves. Social historians, by contrast, remain most focused on unearthing from unpublished sources the voices and lives of the disenfranchised, traditionally construed as lacking secure or any access to formal education or "high culture."[28] While research in recent decades has challenged the assumption that, for instance, a cobbler would not have heard of Tacitus let alone owned the *Annals,* the ghost of such an assumption still lurks in history's interpretive machinery.

Studies within what has come to be called the "social history of ideas," following Peter Gay's coinage in the 1960s, tend to align with one or another of three primary lines of inquiry.[29] At the most theoretical level, scholars such as Roger Chartier and Peter Burke have given us sociologies of knowledge that reveal the ways in which different social worlds constitute, if not determine, the meanings of languages, educational traditions and institutions, information storage and retrieval systems, the production and distribution of books, the practices of reading, the collection and display of cultural artifacts, and the dynamics of knowledge communities.[30] Other social historians of ideas aim to embed specific authors within their everyday worlds, as Gay attempted to do with Enlightenment philosophes, and as many others, especially but not exclusively within the history of science, have done with increasing sophistication in recent years. Mario Biagioli, for instance, famously reframed Galileo as a Medici courtier.[31] Stephen Shapin showed us Robert Boyle and his colleagues contorting to accommodate contemporary expectations for "epistemological decorum" and the character of the independent and thus trustworthy gentleman.[32] Paula Findlen uncovered the prehistory of museums in large domestic collections of early-modern Italy, paradigmatically that of Ulisse Aldrovandi, which became surprisingly inclusive forums for intellectual exchange.[33] All three scholars have taught us that early-modern science as a pursuit, and the particular careers of early-modern natural philosophers, had as much to do with skillful networking as it did with content knowledge. Historians of science are not alone in this approach. Scholars of humanism such as Lauro Martines, Diana Robin, Christopher Celenza, Brian Maxson, and others have revealed the networks connecting the Renaissance republic of letters.[34] Those of us working on intellectual women, moreover, have of necessity wrestled with the ways in which relational forces shaped women's literary possibilities.[35]

The social historians of ideas who adopt a third approach recover broader patterns of book ownership and the reading practices (especially but not exclusively) of nonelites from collections of popular literature and the widest possible selection of archival materials. This third approach most often provides insight into the literary lives of the peasantry, artisans, and the middling sort. An approach favored by *Annalistes,* Albert Labarre's classic study of book ownership in sixteenth-century Amiens exemplifies the empirical riches it can yield.[36]

Each of these modalities has its strengths and to a degree relies on the others, but there have been and continue to be methodological tensions. Not long after Gay coined the phrase "social history of ideas," Robert Darnton issued a stirring manifesto for a methodology that might help reconcile these related but divergent projects.[37] The chasm he saw between the "library" people, exemplified by Gay, and the "archive" people, represented by the annalistes, has narrowed in the ensuing decades. The increasing integration of intellectual and social questions owes much, in fact, to Darnton's own work. Whether finding deep meaning in the ritual execution of cats or reminding us that books may indeed cause revolutions—even if those books were more likely to have been pulp fiction than political philosophy—he models ways to divine what people read, how they read, and sometimes why, toggling back and forth between the individual document and evidence drawn from print culture.[38]

My own study owes the greatest debt to Darnton's anatomy of the mid-eighteenth-century republic of letters through the trove of case files left by a literary-minded police inspector for the book trade, Joseph d'Hémery.[39] Darnton excavates the raw data furnished by d'Hémery's files from a prosopography of the republic's citizens, while also considering the larger problems this citizenry raises: the emergence of the writer as a figure, the conceptual category of "Enlightenment," and the tensions surrounding the act of authorship, especially the constraints and even the violence of patronage systems. Darnton's inspector led him to the thought worlds of many people beyond Voltaire. We meet 501 individuals whom d'Hémery genially stalked, hundreds of men and women who had written at least a line or two for a periodical. If fathers' occupations are taken into account, 19 percent of these writers belonged to the *petites gens.*[40] Fully 70 percent of them belonged to the third estate.[41] Statistically speaking, then, literary work meant more to the middling sort than it did to the nobility in Enlightenment France. Mapping another corner of this world, Darnton has also unearthed impassioned letters written by a bourgeois book collector and fanatical reader of Rousseau to his favorite printer-publisher.[42] In these materials, Darnton reveals that everyday people cared very much about books and authors, even if the lack of peasants reminds us that the ranks of the literate remained comparatively circumscribed throughout the early-modern period.

We certainly have models, then, for giving intellectual and social issues close to equal weight, but instabilities in conceptualization remain. Darnton, for instance, harbored a prejudice against tabulations of book inventories and the generalizations drawn from them. "Cultural objects are not manufactured by the historian but by the people he studies," Darnton chastised. "They give off meaning. They need to be read, not counted."[43] On the one hand, few of us would challenge the notion that statistics can reveal much without careful connection to other sources. On the other hand, Darnton's locution invites historians' continued reliance on evidence susceptible to the literary analysis that Darnton wants—in other words, texts. That reliance, in turn, risks keeping the spotlight on those who left substantial documentary trails, which often means the privileged. Numbers have the distinct advantage of urging us to consider the full range of participants in the history of ideas.

As we continue to amass data, however, we should be aware that the interpretive rubrics within which we work tend still to reproduce older assumptions about the effects of social stratification. One important synthetic study exemplifying this tendency is Roger Chartier's primer to the sociology of knowledge, *The Order of Books.* Chartier states at the outset that "communities of readers" must be understood as dynamic, active, and plural. He speaks eloquently against understanding literary and cultural commitments as "necessarily organized according to pre-existent social divisions," and terms any binary conception of high versus low culture "a mutilated conception of the social."[44] Chartier goes on to insist, "The *same* texts were appropriated by 'popular' readers and other readers more than has been thought."[45] Yet this promising argument for multiplicity soon retrogrades toward binaries. "Readers of more humble social condition," he continues, "were put in possession of books [*aient été mis en possession des livres*] that were not specifically designed for them." He further notes that "inventive and canny bookseller-printers made available to a very large clientele texts that formerly had circulated only in the narrow world of wealth and letters." The passive construction conjures the image of an inert mass on which shrewd pressmen foisted reading material—an image Chartier cannot have intended, as it contravenes his own argument about the active nature of individual reading. Yet he goes on to characterize these men and women as "readers of humble social condition" *(lecteurs d'humble condition)* inhabiting a social space outside "the narrow world of wealth and letters" *(le monde étroit des lettrés fortunés),* which we might also translate "the restricted territory of wealthy, well-read people."[46] We thus return to a socioeconomic opposition: people of "humble condition" versus a world of financial privilege coextensive if not coterminous with the world of intellectual privilege. That binary, in turn, inflects Chartier's characterization of reading practices. We must, he concludes, "understand how the same texts can be differently apprehended, manipulated, and comprehended" by readers who lived outside the gated community of the *lettrés fortunés*.[47] Chartier's participles leave little room for informed, even if divergent and alternative reading, suggesting instead misreading.[48] Despite the disavowals, then, Chartier remains within the ambit of a "high culture" versus "low culture" model.[49] Once his exposition moves from readers to authors and conceptions of the library, moreover, everyday people recede and the erudite return to their usual place of prominence.

Peter Burke's recent contributions to the sociology and anthropology of knowledge also continue to sort complex sets of evidence and otherwise nuanced readings under strangely static conceptual rubrics such as "insider" versus "outsider" communities, and "popular" versus "elite" reading modalities. Such rubrics are even stranger to find here, given that Burke himself changed the field with his two-way model for the movement of cultural forms, including ideas, between more and less socioeconomically privileged groups.[50] Here again, conceptual binaries filter through in unfortunate ways, for instance, in the opposition Burke posits between "practical literacy," useful for getting things done in business, family, church, and government, and the (implicitly impractical) skills necessary for appreciating *bonae litterae*.[51] Armando Petrucci has gone a long way toward pluralizing even this conception literacy, positing an intricate spectrum of reading and writing abilities and an equally diverse range of their potential uses.[52] And scholars have also raised important questions about our definitions of practicality. Lorna Weatherill, for one, argues that our historical subjects might see literary texts no less than games or art as "deeply valued, and thus, in some sense, necessary."[53]

If Burke's conception of practical versus ornamental literacies at least hints at the possibility for more complex shadings of skills and objectives, he nonetheless tethers texts to context-specific assumed values. "What individuals believe to be truth or knowledge is influenced, if not determined, by their social milieu," Burke observes.[54] The argument for influence is unimpeachable, for determinism much less so. Unfortunately the exposition tends toward determinism, in the end a polarity of "academic" knowledge and "alternative knowledges" of the type possessed, for instance, by itinerant healers, Moriscos, and women.[55] Burke then sorts these knowledges further, according to social group: "Intellectuals are masters of some kinds of knowledge, but other fields of expertise or 'know how' are cultivated by such groups as bureaucrats, artisans, peasants, midwives and popular healers," possessors of what he then terms "implicit knowledge."[56]

With "alternative" or "implicit" knowledge versus "dominant" or "academic" knowledge we return to the conceptual binary. Thereafter Burke, like Chartier, moves on to his paradigmatic Renaissance readers. In Burke's case, those readers are Montaigne and Montesquieu.[57]

As pioneers, Darnton, Chartier, and Burke show the road forward while also revealing some of its obstacles. In their different ways, each makes the crucial claim that premodern literary cultures were pluralistic, but each also reveals how difficult it is to capture differences without invoking binaries. Conceptions of "high" and "low" culture keep returning to our research and writing, just when we thought we had modified or even deleted them.

These persistent disjunctures also affect work on the history of consumption, which might be one means of continuing to keep everyday readers in view. Books as goods, however, tend to occupy the margins in this line of inquiry. Vast libraries appear as part of the voracious collecting on the part of a Medici or a d'Este, for instance, in recent studies by Lisa Jardine and Evelyn Welch.[58] Yet books at large do not receive consideration as consumer objects. To learn about books in conjunction with other uses of discretionary income among different social groups, we must turn to rare targeted studies such as that of Lorna Weatherill.[59] Scholars of literary culture and scholars of consumer culture, then, while certainly in conversation, still tend to pursue different questions.

Here again, however, historians of science have made strides in bringing disparate lines of inquiry together. Pamela Smith and Pamela Long form part of a vanguard emphasizing the active roles played by artisans in the rise of the new science, the collaboration of artisans with theoreticians, and the frequency with which individuals had both manual skills and book learning.[60] Intellectual and literary historians should attend more to this work. We know that Galileo both knew Latin and modified a spyglass. Yet we have not actively sought out and analyzed the literary lives of artisans who lived primarily by craftwork, because we still tend to assume that these men and women would not have known Latin, or even been able to read in the vernacular, let alone have felt any desire to purchase translations of Ovid and Josephus—or at least not in numbers sufficient to save us from accusations of studying exceptions.

Scholarship on book culture offers a promising avenue to bring the insights of the history of science concerning artisan-intellectuals into literary domains. Scholars in this field continue to show us the importance of the "print revolution" while directing our attention to the unpredictable relationships between producers, texts, and readers.[61] Especially illuminating for thinking about early-modern literary consumption, Ann Blair has shown us an extensive community of scholars who devised new search, storage, and retrieval methods to capitalize on the early-modern "information explosion."[62] Turning to an even more diverse group of people, William Sherman brings into sharp relief the specific passages that drew English readers' attention, even if his reliance on marginalia limits somewhat the range of texts he could use.[63]

Again, however, synthetic assessments have not caught up with empirical studies. Recent comprehensive treatments of early-modern book history do situate literary culture as a marketplace and emphasize its diversity. Yet they still rehearse older models of readerly segregation by arguing that, excepting the broad readership of a few best sellers such as the *Decameron, Don Quixote,* or *Amadis de Gaulle,* the erudite and wealthy read scholarship and literature, whereas nonelites consumed devotional material and tales of "marvels."[64] It is perhaps small wonder that our historical shorthand seems so impervious to change, given that scholars who have developed highly nuanced conceptions of literacy, among them Armando Petrucci, still let conceptions of the broadest patterns of book ownership stand unqualified; even here, we are told that the bulk of reading material in circulation pertained to religion, with school texts and vernacular translations of the classics coming in a distant second, and other genres filtering in with increasingly meager showings down to the rarest specialist Latin works on medicine, rhetoric, and law.[65] While print runs have significance, they should not set the parameters for discussions of early-modern encounters with texts as much as they still do.

Archives furnish contrary evidence for any generalization we want to make, including old claims about readers' tastes. We have learned a great deal from scholars working in the Italian archives about the literary range of most social groups, if not about the particular benefits they derived from the purchases their household inventories reveal. Christian Bec has offered us a magisterial account of book ownership in fifteenth- and sixteenth-century Florence, finding the most voracious consumers among the mercantile and citizen orders.[66] More recently, as noted earlier, art historian Renata Ago has drawn on household inventories in seventeenth-century Rome to illuminate not only the art, luxury goods, musical instruments, and books collected by an impressive swath of society, which again shows the middling sort to be the most consistently engaged in cultural collecting if not (owing to their more limited means) the owners of the largest collections.[67] Isabella Cecchini takes a similar approach in a multidimensional study of Venetian inventories 1511–1633, though her primary concern remains art.[68] We also have the meticulous research of Susan Connell and Marino Zorzi, who used inventories to unearth patterns of book circulation in Venice during the fifteenth and sixteenth centuries—patterns that once again reveal literary passions centering in the mercantile and citizen ranks.[69]

This is an exciting moment, then, to join conversations at the crossroads of social and intellectual history that now span eras and geopolitical contexts while continuing to question access to and interest in literary material. "Great books had plebeian readers," insists Jonathan Rose as he introduces his magisterial analysis of book ownership and readership in nineteenth- and early twentieth-century England.[70] Some of the sources that bolster Rose's claim, for instance, the records of mutual improvement societies and libraries' extensive borrowing records, do not exist for the Renaissance era. Yet there are plenty of evidentiary trails early modernists and Italianists can follow and have followed to rethink our persistent assumptions about early-modern readers and listeners. Indeed, pioneering works of micro-history got us started long ago. Carlo Ginzburg found in the Inquisitional records a sixteenth-century Friulan miller who was also a keen reader and formulated a bizarre, idiosyncratic cosmology on this basis of his reading.[71] Duccio Balestracci showed us the "Renaissance in the fields" of fifteenth-century Tuscan peasants who, inspired by the record-keeping mania of the era, paid notaries to chronicle their family histories alongside their business transactions.[72] More recently and speaking, like Rose, as an intellectual historian, Christopher Celenza has urged scholars of Renaissance humanism to learn from micro-historians how to embed ideas more deeply in their social and cultural contexts, as well as to reconsider the traditional boundaries drawn between "high" and "low" culture.[73]

While retaining the traditional emphasis on textual material, David Ruderman and Nancy Siraisi have innovatively pointed to the different cultural positions that even educated men occupied when they moved outside their areas of specialization. Ruderman and Siraisi show us rabbis and physicians, respectively, inhabiting literary middle zones. When they dealt outside their areas of mastery to discuss (in the case of rabbis) scientific matters or (in the case of physicians) popular history, news, and divination, these ostensible members of "high" culture inhabited far less exalted readerly and writerly spaces.[74] But even here the problematic terminology remains, as well as the emphasis on career intellectuals, rather than amateur reading or collecting. Neither scholar delves into their protagonists' family backgrounds or connects these particular cases to broader sociocultural trends.

Everyday Renaissances dispenses altogether with conceptions of "high" and "low" culture, as well as integrating these two disciplines' methodologies and their characteristic sets of evidence. This is a history of ideas drawn principally from sources dear to social historians: wills, household inventories, and account books. Our ensemble of protagonists allows us to think about intellectual life outside the realm of notable minds, on the one hand, and broad statistics on the other. Drawing at once on discursive documents (testaments, diary entries, and of course some printed works) and inventories that yield numerical data, this book finds traces of learning everywhere—traces susceptible at once to social, intellectual, and material analysis. While my treatment of inventories does lie open to Darnton's charge of counting more than revealing reading practices, by connecting these numbers to the literary priorities evident in more discursive sources, I do ultimately arrive at books' social and literary significance.

In toggling between objects, texts, and meanings, *Everyday Renaissances* engages several topical literatures beyond the social history of ideas. Given the emphasis on books and learning, I interact with recent work on the vernacularization of humanism. As so many of my protagonists are physicians, the history of medicine remains another crucial frame of reference. And analyzing intellectual honor and related claims to cultural legitimacy brings me to interact with scholarship on the family, in particular with recent studies of social mobility. While the vast majority of previous research along my lines of inquiry has been done by Anglophone scholars, I hope that this study's attention to work by Italian and, to a lesser degree, French historians may help spark new conversations at the interstices of social, intellectual, and cultural history in larger European academic circles.

The subjects of this study cannot be termed humanists by any definition currently available. My protagonists were not Kristellerian philologists who had full command of grammar, rhetoric, history, poetry, and moral philosophy; nor did they follow closely "in the footsteps of the ancients" by appropriating classical Latin style and usage in the specific ways that Ronald Witt has shown humanists doing.[75] Many of my protagonists would not even fit within the more pliable definition of humanism as a principal commitment to the classical tradition, ornately rhetorical self-presentation, and privileging of original sources employed by Anthony Grafton, Craig Kallendorf, Jill Kraye, Adam Shear, and others.[76] A few of the more voracious book collectors and some of the physicians in this study might pass these more general criteria, but only just. My conception of the significance of the literary, however, and the value attached to it does engage work on humanism in a general way. The Venetian men and women we will meet became members of humanism's audience, belonging to the lineage of the literary by extension. Even those who had Latin, as we will see, never felt entirely confident of their membership in the humanist community. What scholars of humanism as such stand to gain from the present study, however, is a better sense of the scope and impact of humanist rhetoric in convincing contemporaries to value the literary.

In turning to humanism's audiences, I follow recent work on the vernacularization of literary culture. James Hankins examined one paradigmatic fifteenth-century humanist, Leonardo Bruni, working in Italian no less than in Latin—a clear indication, as Hankins demonstrated, that Bruni aimed to bring classical moral philosophy to those who could only read Italian and in so doing tap the considerable vernacular market.[77] I also benefit from Brian Maxson's decentering of elite producers in his analysis of the degrees of humanism exhibited by those who did not publish.[78] While retaining as a defining feature the commitment to the classical tradition, Maxson posits an important distinction between what he terms "literary humanists," producers of complex works in humanist genres as well as the most ardent consumers of humanists' publications, and "social humanists," by which he indicates men and women who engaged the new learning tangentially, often through contact with more ardent devotees instead of independent intellectual endeavor. Some social humanists had demonstrable contact with writers, scholars, and philologists through correspondence; others put their Latin competency in the service of the Florentine diplomatic corps as orators. Maxson abjures binaries, noting that many individuals displayed characteristics of both types. Yet "social humanism" still does not quite work for my protagonists, many of whom did not have connections to career humanists. At a more fundamental level, moreover, I resist retaining classicism as the benchmark of participation in literary culture, as it excludes too many people who participated by means of "modern" literature. And while Maxson makes a compelling case that humanists changed conceptions of merit in political culture to emphasize intellectual and literary capabilities, his focus on governmental politics, as he concedes, necessarily keeps the spotlight on men, patricians, and the wealthy.[79]

How can we assess Renaissance literary life more fully? Lynn Enterline has shown us a new world of literary consumption and humanistic priorities by examining grammar-school graduates in Elizabethan England.[80] Interweaving schoolbooks and pedagogical treatises with Shakespeare's plays and poetry, as well as the works of his contemporaries, Enterline demonstrates that humanist pronouncements about the value of the liberal arts for creating "gentlemen" went in different directions when appropriated by students, many of whom (including Shakespeare) had artisanal and mercantile social backgrounds. Following these lines of inquiry, I focus on the issues of humanistic demand and consumption, from the extensive literary ruminations of physicians to a pharmacist's wife who stipulated in her will that her husband must spend no fewer than five years teaching their son to read well.

Given the prominence of physicians in this study, the history of medicine holds a central place in the analysis. In approaching medical culture, I build on work in the social history of medicine, particularly the studies of Venetian physicians by Richard Palmer and the wider assessment of physicians' roles in Renaissance Italy by Gianna Pomata and Katherine Park.[81] I also draw on a comparatively recent line of inquiry: early-modern cultures of healing, which spanned different social and occupational groups, among which studies by David Gentilcore and Mary Lindemann have been most helpful.[82] In emphasizing physicians' literary ambitions, my principal model is Nancy Siraisi's *History, Medicine and the Traditions of Renaissance Learning.*[83] Siraisi has redirected our attention to physicians' literary passions, above all in the field of history, beyond their particular contributions to medical knowledge or practice. *Everyday Renaissances,* taking a cue from Siraisi's work on humanistic physicians as well as the research that she, Douglas Biow, and George McClure have done on humanist conceptions of the professions, moves further into the archives to highlight the social and professional stakes of physicians' interdisciplinary endeavors.[84]

In considering the connections between learning and socioprofessional mobility, I aim to modify our understanding of family strategies as primarily concerned with economic and marital issues. Studies of social mobility and family history in Venice continue to follow models such as James Davis's *A Venetian Family and Its Fortune* that focus on the accumulation and conservation of wealth, as well as marriage strategies.[85] In making education and literary cachet a part of the calculations, I draw inspiration first from Maxson, who also posits that intellectual and literary endeavors catalyzed socioeconomic mobility. Most of his humanistic correspondents and unheralded orators constitute new figures for us to consider, men who did not begin life primed for election to government service, even if they belonged to the patriciate or enjoyed considerable wealth.[86] Maxson's argument for educational social mobility in a more dramatic sense, however, rests primarily on the example of Bartolomeo Scala.[87] To be sure, Scala proves the point. But as we work to change paradigms in social history, we will need evidence beyond a few well-known individuals, who can always be dismissed (even if misguidedly) as exceptional cases.

While rooted in the eighteenth-century Ottoman world, Dana Sajdi's analysis of the historical and biographical writing of an eighteenth-century Damascene barber offers another source of encouragement for considering the connection between education, writing, and social mobility.[88] Sajdi's concept of "nouveau literacy" encapsulates the entrance of nonelites into academic activity across the Ottoman world and the social mobility they often enjoyed thereafter. Explicating the cultural legitimacy of everyday

Venetian testators and the city's bibliophilia, an honorable pathology that physicians had in a particularly acute form, I find, like Sajdi, literary endeavors and social advancement to be mutually sustaining across a wide spectrum of people. Meritocracy was not just an ideal in the republic of letters; it formed an important part of some families' strategies.

EVERYDAY RENAISSANCES IN VENICE

This study has an itinerary with two major destinations. Part I maps the worlds of literary consumption and aspiration through two chapters that explore the different paths to books and learning, honor, and status revealed by my wider sets of archival evidence. Part II turns from the macroscopic to the microscopic, considering individual approaches to cultural legitimacy through three narrative case studies.

Who owned reading material or spoke of educational goals? What types of books did middling-sort Venetians have in their houses? How did families understand and attempt to transmit their cultural legitimacy? These are the fundamental questions addressed in Part I. Chapter 1 analyzes patterns of Venetian book ownership. As we will see, physicians were the most voracious, one might also say the most anxious, literary collectors. But medical doctors were not alone in their passion for texts. Nor do the genres collectors emphasize mesh with models of socioeconomic divisions or professional libraries. Venetian literary consumers of all social stations collected a variety of reading material. Inventories tell an important story about cultural priorities, but in a necessarily laconic way. Fortunately, we have other avenues to explore for seeking out the literary lives of Venice's reading public. In concluding this first chapter, I consider classical and literary naming practices as one possibility. Chapter 2 continues the thought, turning to Venetians' explicit statements about their ethical, bibliographic, and pedagogical commitments in their final wills and testaments, expressions that I am terming "testamentary humanism." By this I do not mean that everyday Venetians imitated some entrenched humanist practice of writing the testament; there was no such practice. Indeed, many card-carrying humanists did not pen or dictate wills that reveal their literary inclinations. Instead, "testamentary humanism" describes the practice of everyday Venetians, often those who did not have a humanist's access to other forms of written expression, who took advantage of the discursive potential of the testament to articulate their literary, bibliographical, pedagogical, or philosophical commitments. In making these bibliographic, educational, and ethical bequests, our Venetians reveal a concern about securing an honorable reputational afterlife that may also have inspired a few notable humanists to bequeath their vast literary collections for "public" use.[89] This book's protagonists did not as a rule have the resources for this sort of elaborate cultural patronage, but they could form libraries that extended beyond devotional and occupational volumes; some also wrote or dictated wills that made literary departures.

Physicians dominate the ranks both of book owners and those who exploited the literary potential of the testament. In seeking answers to why that should have been the case, Part II anatomizes medical doctors' quest for cultural legitimacy through a triptych of case studies. Chapter 3 explores the quest for literary cachet through close examination of the life and career of Nicolò Massa (1485–1569) and the networks emanating from the sodalities to which he belonged, especially Venice's College of Physicians. Massa and his colleagues reveal a common aim of securing humanistic recognition for the profession. Massa's print campaigns, his library, and his ornately rhetorical wills (especially his forty-page draft will) all represented him as a self-made man of letters. In this, his priorities meshed with those of his colleagues and college, whose orations and print publications defended medicine as a liberal art from the disparagement of literary humanists.

But the value of books and education was not always so instrumental. If Massa and some of his colleagues used their learning pragmatically as cultural capital, Francesco Longo (1506–1576) redirects our attention to cultural legitimacy's more idealistic dimensions. Chapter 4 offers a close reading of Longo's two ethical testaments, drawing out their social, intellectual, and literary meanings and recovering what can be known of the life circumstances shaping them from Longo's matriculation records at the University of Padua, as well as other private family documents and the records of the convent of Corpus Domini, where his daughter Virginia took her vows. Longo enjoyed some recognition in the medical community in his lifetime, but he held a place several rungs below Massa on that professional ladder. He published nothing, so far as we know, nor did he hold any civic offices, and his resources were just sufficient for his family's needs. In his two loquacious and philosophical final testaments, Longo made repeated and extensive references to the ancient Persian king Artaxerxes, carefully divided his "Latin, Greek and vernacular books" among his children, and dispensed crash courses in moral philosophy as ethical bequests. In these small textual monuments, he immortalized himself not as a physician but as a man who belonged to the world of letters and possessed a philosophical mind. Longo's self-conception as a moral philosopher, irrespective of his particular job description, and his deference to general Stoic precepts and modes of reasoning situate this physician within a cultural paradigm that Pierre Hadot finds exemplified by Marcus Aurelius.[90]

But if one of the distinctive practices of Hadot's Marcus Aurelius was the emperor's turn to writing as a spiritual exercise, then another Venetian physician, while less overtly philosophical in his expressions than Longo, exhibits even more kinship with this ancient model. Alberto Rini (d. 1599) articulated in his own way how much the literary Renaissance mattered to someone outside the elite of the republic of letters. Chapter 5 offers a close reading of two manuscript treasures, Rini's *giornali,* which record both his daily life and the life of his mind. Once again, we see a physician who, like Longo, left no traces on the print record but was anything but intellectually dormant. Rini's *giornali* detail not only his routine expenditures but also his bouts of note taking at sermons, his recipe collections, his mania for copying chronicles, his appreciation and purchases of art, and his pride in making new additions to the family's growing library of (nonmedical) books. Like Longo, Rini had a passion for culture and education. And Rini created a monument of himself in much the same manner as Longo did. While others, for instance, his colleague Tommaso Rangone, chose commemoration in bronze and in their professional guise, Rini and Longo preferred fragile paper and the personae of *letterati* and philosophers. In choosing what Matthew Lundin has eloquently termed "paper memory" for his posterity, Rini, like Longo, reveals a literary excitement and optimism, even in moments of despair.[91] Even for uncelebrated Venetians, confidence, satisfaction, and even social honor might have to do with the mind less than the wealth or occupational prestige.

In the aggregate, our 147 book collectors and humanistic testators, with our three insistently rhetorical physicians, help us think afresh about the literary Renaissance. We have long befriended behemoths of erudition who enjoyed unrestricted access to Parnassus. We are getting better acquainted with professionals who formed at least discipline-specific libraries, adding perhaps some art or antiquities to ornament their *studioli.* And our familiarity with vernacular readers reaching for prayer books, romances, and news has also deepened. But as we think of these general categories of people and the patterns of their interaction with the written word, let us also think about interstitial cases, letting their sometimes surprising degrees of access to materials, their wide-ranging interests, and their complex aspirations challenge our interpretive models. I hope this book will encourage us to keep on the lookout for provisional literati like those whom we meet here: wives of goldsmiths harboring copies of Lucan and Josephus, professionals desperate to be (or be seen as) literary, and even the occasional retailer borrowing works of Greek philosophy. These men and women can be useful guides to the early-modern republic of letters in their own right; at the least, they sharpen our image of that imaginary republic's very real audiences, and its aspiring citizens.

PART I

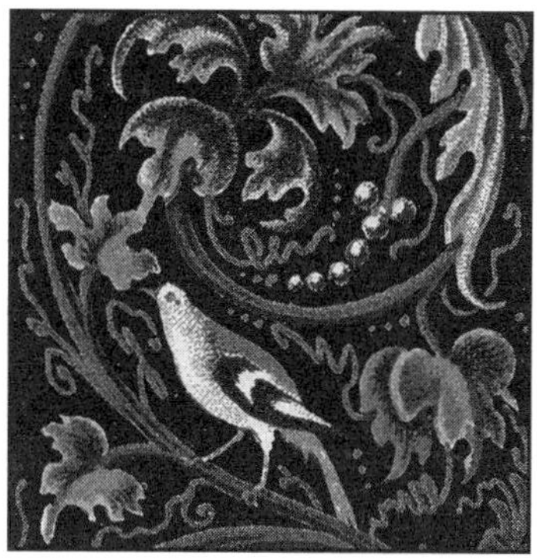

CHAPTER 1

VENICE'S READING PUBLIC

Venetians cared about books and learning. If older scholarship on Renaissance literary culture in Italian cities privileged the erudite manuscripts and printed volumes of famous humanists, newer approaches are illuminating vibrant book cultures formed by other social and professional groups. Brian Maxson has most recently excavated fifteenth-century correspondence and orations from the Florentine archives to reveal one hundred individuals engaging with humanism in tangential ways that situate them, in his formulation, as "social" rather than "literary" humanists.[1] Joining Maxson in reconsidering humanism's scope and impact, even if departing from his emphasis on Florentine political culture, this chapter offers its own reassessment of literary life, more loosely affiliated to humanistic priorities and in the context of Venice.

The lagoon city's intellectual and artistic culture has been mapped by scholars as diverse as Margaret King, Craig Kallendorf, and Patricia Brown, who show us in rich detail the experiences, contributions, and collections of elites.[2] But we can find more everyday Renaissances in Venetian households, following historians of material culture in analyzing inventories, while also seeking the literary in other sources, especially final wills and testaments. Inventories and testaments cannot tell us everything we want to know about the early-modern reading public, but they bring us closer to literary possessions and sometimes to the motives that spurred individuals to acquire books.

In these archival records, we find at least provisional answers to the sorts of questions we asked but could not ultimately answer about an individual like messer Francesco, the retailer interested in Greek philosophy, whose intellectual life remains accessible to us in only one act of book borrowing. If we had a sense of the volumes he kept at home or any indication that he bequeathed books or art to friends and relatives—even if we did not have firm numbers for his collection or know their titles—we could make better guesses about what he really wanted with those manuscripts. Indeed, we will return periodically to messer Francesco in this and Chapter 2. The apparent mismatch between a retailer's ordinary social and professional position and his esoteric readerly interests makes him a useful point of reference as we explore Venetians' different paths to, uses of, and future plans for books and education.

In the course of reading 1,227 household inventories and 3,005 sixteenth-century wills, I located 147 Venetian men and women of the urban middle ranks who engaged the Renaissance in direct ways. A representative cross section of society, these individuals are nonetheless the tip of the iceberg that was Venetian cultural life. Books were not top priorities in household inventories, whose principal object was to assess possessions with the most significant cash value, from real estate and furniture to household ornaments, art, coins, and jewels. Nor did testators usually have the time or energy to reflect on their reading, philosophies, or educational plans for their children.[3] And notaries faced stern injunctions from governing bodies and authors of best practices to restrain their clients from indulging in tangential or superfluous reflections that might create ambiguities or opportunities for conflict among beneficiaries.[4] The Venetians seeking cultural legitimacy whom we encounter through inventories and testaments, then, become historically significant not for their numbers but for the evidence they furnish of literary interests in society's middle ranks, and for the hopes suggested and expressed in relation to those interests. We know from many scholars that urban Italians enjoyed access to education and literacy.[5] Continued contact with books and learning evinced the honor of book owners and testators, and offered possibilities for social motion in future generations. The everyday Renaissances taking place in Venice's artisanal, mercantile, and professional households corroborate our growing sense that humanistic culture had diverse audiences. In fact, these everyday renaissances teach us that humanistic culture, far from being the sole concern of either the economic or the cultural aristocracy, may have meant even more to people living outside the republic of letters than to those who enjoyed comfortable places at the center.

VENETIAN INVENTORIES: THE BIG PICTURE

As many scholars have shown, household inventories help us recover artifacts of culture in ways that other documents, even other archival sources, cannot. We owe a particular debt to three scholars who have modeled the use of inventories for surveying the most prominent features of Venice's intellectual and literary topography: Susan Connell's work on fifteenth-century Venetian book lists; Isabella Cecchini's analysis of sixteenth-century Venetians' collections of art, musical instruments, and books; and Marino Zorzi's analysis of Cinquecento Venetian book ownership.[6]

Connell targeted the wills, account books, and sale records housed in the archives of the Procuratori di San Marco looking for book lists, which ultimately revealed eighteen book owners who died between 1345 and 1480. Of the sixteen cases she found in which records specify the owner's status or profession, middle-rank owners predominate: she located six patrician book collectors, but two lawyers and one other man in a civil profession, five parish priests, one merchant mariner, one physician, and even one engraver. Cecchini, giving pride of place to art, nonetheless considered ownership of books in her analysis of 1,390 posthumous inventories, predominantly relating to owners who had died intestate, recorded by officials of the Giudici del Proprio between 1511 and 1615.[7] According to Cecchini's grouping, the social sectors best represented were patricians (14 percent of the sample), *cittadini* (a category problematically framed to encompass merchants of every type and members of all the professions, 14 percent), and artisans-shopkeepers (37 percent). Books only appear in this set of inventories between 3 and 7 percent of the time, but when they do emerge, we most often find them in possession of *cittadini*. Spanning the whole century, patrician inventories mention books between 7 and 9 percent of the time, and artisan-shopkeepers' 3 to 7 percent; by contrast, *cittadini* inventories include books in 10–19 percent of cases.[8]

The image of Venice's reading public we get from Connell and Cecchini reinforces the notion that book culture's strongest adherents were men and women in the middle ranks of society. Yet these studies make it difficult to gauge literary culture in the later Renaissance, or get a closer look at owners. Connell teaches us only about the fifteenth century. And Cecchini offers neither numbers of volumes nor any particular titles. Questions about the sixteenth century also remain unresolved in Cecchini's research, since more than half of her inventories (773) are dated 1610–1615.

The world of books in Cinquecento Venice emerges with the most detail in the work of Marino Zorzi. Looking both for numbers and types of volumes owned between 1511 and 1600, Zorzi sought out a larger sample than we find in Connell or Cecchini. Surveying 730 inventories dated 1527–1599 from a notarial miscellany under the jurisdiction of the Cancelleria Inferiore and 207 cases from the Giudici di Petizion dated 1580–1600, he found 937 cases of book owners who represent, once again, a broad cross section of the urban population. Unlike Cecchini's inventories, which suggest at best a 7 percent rate of book ownership in this city, Zorzi finds that between 10 percent and 15 percent of Venetian households harbored books.[9]

In seeking a still sharper image of Venice's reading public, I assembled a larger group of 1,227 inventories, following Zorzi in giving special attention to the Cancelleria Inferiore series but including more inventories from the Giudici di Petizion. Whereas he considered 207 inventories from this series, I have added more than 500. I have also incorporated a few inventories from the records housed at the Archivio IRE, a collection focused on the history of charitable institutions in which we find inventories connected to pious bequests. Beyond casting a wider evidentiary net, I give the most consideration to literary collecting among groups usually relegated to margins. Focused on the concept of a "library," for instance, Zorzi gives little consideration to smaller book collections or artisanal, mercantile, and professional owners.[10] In general terms, my inventories reveal similar patterns of ownership, in particular the frequency with which professionals collected literary material. But artisans play stronger roles here than the secretaries and lawyers who loom large in other studies do. And physicians emerge as the most consistent and omnivorous collectors.

Taking to heart Robert Darnton's warning that inventories can make false promises to the social historian of ideas, this chapter details the particularities of texts owned specifically within the middling ranks and suggests their possible meanings. These suggestions get closer scrutiny in Chapter 2, which examines the bibliographic and intellectual commitments signaled in final testaments, subjecting this discursive evidence to more literary analysis in search of answers to the question of what benefits books and learning brought those who possessed them.

But who were the Venetians in a position to read and own books in the first place? Debates rage concerning early-modern literacy rates and the suitable sources and methods for determining them. Situating conservative and optimistic claims as a range, we may imagine full vernacular literacy in Italian urban centers between a pessimistic 23 percent combined literacy and a rate of 60 percent male literacy.[11] In the case of Venice, we may incline with some security toward the optimistic end of this spectrum, given the city's outstanding pedagogical amenities and extensive book trade. Even discounting the instruction in convents and monasteries, as well as private tutors and other forms of homeschooling, at any given moment in the sixteenth century this territory of approximately 150,000 souls boasted more than eight hundred formal instructors at the elementary and grammar level.[12] Even during the crisis of the later sixteenth century, when pressures from the Index nudged printers to prioritize devotional material and to exercise more caution with risky literary material, Venice nonetheless remained a print capital of Europe.[13] More than one hundred printers worked in the city, generating books by the tens of thousands each year. Girolamo Scotto (1505–1572), for instance, printed more than eight hundred editions in three decades at midcentury, meaning that he alone brought something on the order of eight thousand books into circulation during only part of his career—an impressive number, even if not all these volumes were intended for the Venetian market.[14]

The evidence of Venetian book ownership offered here furnishes a minimalist image of cultural life in this vibrant city. Much as with tabulating literacy rates, the scholar of book ownership must rely on documents whose creators were inconsistent in their procedures, meaning that only a fraction of references can be incorporated into the analysis. I have counted only those inventories that referred to texts, leaving aside mention of "books" that might have been for reading but might also have been account books. Sometimes the assessors included the titles of volumes they found scattered throughout households and in rare cases assessors provided a full book inventory. More often, however, assessors wrote only a number, and that usually some general indication such as "about 40 books" or the slightly more helpful "53 books, 20 pertaining to the humanities, 30 law books, and three prayer books." Usually, however, assessors give more vague indications, for instance, "some printed books" or "a few texts for reading." The level of detail depended on the assessor, as well as desires and finances of those who called for the inventory.

Of my 1,227 inventories, 221 (18 percent) mention books for reading specifically. I have further refined this group with the aim of screening out owners of the odd prayer book or missal, which might be evidence of literacy but not necessarily of literary interests. Accordingly, and following one common procedure among book historians and scholars of material culture, I set the minimum number of five items to count as a collection.[15] For purposes of making the most reliable comparisons, I focused on those inventories that satisfied two further conditions: the owner's occupation was either indicated or could be determined from internal evidence and the assessors either evaluated the texts numerically or provided an itemized list of authors or titles.

My hyperrestricted group of book owners comprises 101 individuals, 34 patricians but 67 other men and women engaged in a variety of urban occupations. Thus far, the finding meshes well with the image of Venetian book owners offered by Marino Zorzi, as well as the collectors of Amiens as studied by Labarre, and those of Florence as they appear in Christian Bec's surveys.[16] But our slightly different sets of data offer predictably different results—not wildly so but significantly. Of the 937 sixteenth-century inventories surveyed by Zorzi, at most 15 percent indicated the presence of books.[17] By contrast, the set of inventories I analyzed noted books, and specifically literary texts, in 18 percent of cases. Mapping these general distributions onto a locality whose population approached 150,000, even a 3 percent difference could mean thousands of readers.

As is common in studies of book ownership, the clerical and legal professions are well represented: I located thirteen clergymen, as well as fourteen lawyers and secretaries. But the marketplace looms larger here. Even Zorzi found that 40 percent of book owners were *cittadini* and only 5 percent retail merchants or artisans.[18] By contrast, 28 percent of my book owners fall into the latter two categories. Our retailer messer Francesco begins to seem less an oddity and more a representative case in his commerce with literary material.

As neither Cecchini nor Zorzi broke down *cittadini* owners by specific status or profession, we cannot know how patterns of collecting might appear in their samples. Looking at my own *cittadini* by profession, the medical field asserted itself with force: Eleven physicians emerge as strong literary collectors, and another seven health practitioners, pharmacists and barber surgeons, joined them. Taken together, those affiliated with medicine constitute 27 percent of book owners in my survey. Given that medical practitioners were a micro-fraction of the population at large, they are dramatically overrepresented here.

Before making a closer quantitative assessment of patterns in Venetian book collecting, it will be useful to think qualitatively. There are many interesting collectors whom I could not incorporate into the quantitative analysis because they fell outside the parameters I established (five volumes minimum) or, more often, because assessors gave vague estimates of the books ("a few," "some," "many") that could not be rendered numerically. Yet we miss much if we discount them altogether, as scholars analyzing inventories tend to do with cases that cannot fit in their tables. These more assorted owners make their own statements about the diversity of Venice's reading public and its interests.

"VARIOUS" BOOKS FOR READING

It is a dictum of book history that when we find households with only one or two books, those volumes tended to be for prayer. On the whole, the Venetian men and women I found fit this general pattern. Yet exceptions appear as well. Bernardo Zonca, a carpenter, owned only one volume, but that happened to be Dante's *Commedia.*[19] A woman called Catharina Raffono owned one work by Ovid and the popular *Doctrinale* (a compilation of Ovidian material), as well as "one other book in the vernacular," all of which she ultimately bequeathed to a metalworker and his wife.[20] We might consider Raffono's choice of recipients for these texts surprising, but Venetian artisans with very few books of their own sometimes displayed literary tastes. Vincenzo di Francesco, for instance, owned only two volumes; one of them was the epistles of the Evangelists, and the other Ariosto's *Satires.*[21] Another book owner, identified as Antonio the perfumer, harbored three books, but these were not (or at least not all) prayer books, which assessors consistently characterized as such. Instead, the scribe noted Antonio's books as being "of various kinds."[22]

These literary-minded artisans militate against the assumption that even tiny collections would have been devotional in nature, indicating at best marginal contact with the world of letters. First of all, as Virginia Reinburg and others have shown, prayer books had pedagogical and aesthetic no less than the spiritual value; so, we should not assume that owners engaged devotional material only for the uses suggested by its genre.[23] Beyond that important argument, however, we also regularly encounter men and women who owned very few volumes but nonetheless evinced inclinations to literature.[24]

When assessors indicated "various" *(diversi)* volumes, even if they did not specify numbers or titles, they were looking at topically if not numerically expansive collections. Instances of this characterization bring us again cases of literary collecting among the lower orders. *Diversi* as a term denotes breadth, but assessors also tended to use this adjective in conjunction with other modifiers indicating varied reading material. For example, we learn that the jewelers Zuanne de Torre and Sabastiano Usnaghi owned "various printed books" *(libri diversi a stampa)* and an ironworker, Pietro son of Andrea, harbored "an assortment of books for reading" *(diversi libri da lezer).*[25] Girolamo Corner, a goldsmith, may not have been much of a reader himself, but he had acquired "various books for his son's use."[26] Even occupational interests might have prompted metalworkers such as these to own texts on metallurgy or, particularly in the case of jewelers and goldsmiths, even classical and modern literature that might furnish descriptions of figures or scenes with which to adorn the objects they created for clients. But the characterizations "books for reading" and "books for his son's use" also suggest that whatever the assessors found struck them as, in the one case, literature and, in the other, schoolbooks. The presence of schoolbooks in an artisanal household hints strongly at educational ambitions for the new generation.

Some artisans formed substantial libraries. We will examine particular instances in detail hereafter, but it is worth pointing out now that the characterization "various books" included both the collections of artisans and those of Venetians in the highest social and income brackets. The libraries of the patricians Nicolò Dolfin, Alvise Gradenigo, and Pietro Gritti were characterized as "various" in nature, but with further specifications of Latin, Greek, and Italian texts and, in one case, an assortment valued at ten ducats.[27] To be sure, this collection paled in comparison to the century's largest. Marin Sanudo's library had grown to sixty-five hundred volumes by 1530, estimating an average value of 1.4 ducats per volume; one gets a sense of true bibliographic luxury.[28] Still, even Gritti's modest library was worth about three months' wages for a skilled craftsman.[29] Other owners of "various" books, moreover, were men whose professions would have necessitated a subject-specific library, such as the ducal secretary Leonardo Masser, the notary Sebastiano Bordonio, the priest Steffano Pozzo, and two lawyers, Giacomo Grataruol and Steffano di Cerchieri.[30] Assessors also used the term *alcuni* (some) to describe book collections. This term may have indicated fewer texts or less varied subject matter than those characterized as "diversi," but not necessarily. Owners of "some" volumes ranged from patricians such as Zuanne Alvise Bragadin and Hortensio Mulo, to a merchant named Christoffolo Vento and three men who had surnames but no titles, indicating that they were probably retail merchants or higher artisans.[31]

Inventories also sometimes assessed books by way of the containers in which they were found. In this case, too, the number of books is impossible to estimate, especially as contemporary art shows books sharing space with other objects in trunks, shelves, and display furniture.[32] However, when assessors mentioned cases, chests, and cabinets "full of books," they indicated a substantial number of volumes. Holders of books that filled at least one *cassa* or *forzier* include, once again, a wide range of people. We find patricians such as Benedetto Superantio and priests like Paolo Signa. But we also meet the linen merchant Francesco de Maphei and a woman named Maria Vinciverre whom the assessors gave no honorific, indicating that she was probably the widow of an artisan.[33] In a few instances, assessors offered more detail. We learn that the physician Francesco Livello's books filled one full "chest" and one "little chest," and were mostly medical texts, but he also had a copy of Boccaccio.[34] A man named Giacomo Pantaleo, termed "spettabile" and thus probably a higher artisan or merchant, owned "a bag full of books" in Italian and Latin. Bernardino Redaldi, probably a pharmacist, had a substantial library. Redaldi's books filled nine regular chests, one little chest, and a *scrigno* (small box for storage), as well as covering the surface of a bench.[35] Book lovers are forever running out of shelf space. But it is remarkable that a pharmacist apparently undistinguished in social or professional terms owned such an array of texts.

I emphasize the collections of artisans and retail merchants at the outset to underscore the utility of pursuing recent lines of inquiry concerning the intellectual and cultural experiences and contributions of nonelites. Scholars such as Pamela Smith have demonstrated that "embodied" knowledge earned respect from those specializing in textual or "abstract" knowledge by the sixteenth century, if not already by the fifteenth.[36] We are also coming to grips with the interchange of these knowledges between groups and within individuals. In the latter case, we need only think of Albrecht Dürer or Benevenuto Cellini. Beyond seeing that artisans' expertise held an honorable place in early-modern textual and scientific culture, thanks to the spadework of James Amelang, we even have a broad checklist of and model for analyzing European artisans' autobiographical writing.[37] Yet synthetic works treating artisans themselves, let alone broader works of intellectual history, have yet to incorporate these trends effectively into their arguments. Even as sophisticated a survey as James Farr's frames artisans' education exclusively in terms of practical skills and devotes no consideration to their writing, book collecting, or literary reading.[38] Whether social or intellectual historians, attending to the presence of artisans diversifies our conception of cultural life.

These artisans might have read their books for pleasure, or bought them in the hopes of encouraging the education of their children; they might also have displayed them in their shops as marks of respectability or occupational credibility. As Pamela Smith notes, artisans and those associated with advanced learning often exchanged knowledge in what she calls "trading zones." Book learning gave the artisan participant more common ground, and possibly more leverage, with their learned collaborators. It is certainly clear from the most famous cases of notable artisans with book learning that their literary competence enhanced their cultural portfolios. In addition to a Dürer or Cellini, we could also point to the renowned Florentine humanist Matteo Palmieri, who also plied the trade of a pharmacist.[39] From Patrick Wallis, too, we have learned much about the importance of display in the marketplace, especially for pharmacists, but the same would have applied to jewelers, carvers, artists, and for that matter even glassmakers and ceramicists.[40] That display might have enhanced both the physical spaces of shops and the products themselves. In the world of ceramics, for instance, we see considerable cultural ambition in a case such as the majolica painter Nicola da Urbino, who included not only classical scenes but also Petrarchan verse on his creations, along with his signature.[41] Artisans, no less than their patrons, surely had aesthetic and literary investments in such material, but they also benefited from conveying an idea of cultural value and "classiness." As Christian Bec observed long ago, Florentine mercantile readers of the early Renaissance tended to leave reading material lying around in the most trafficked areas of their houses and businesses, doing so as a form of visual ennoblement, advertising their belonging to the ranks of the educated.[42]

What most deserves emphasis here, however, is the range of materials we have seen in artisanal and mercantile households. We have metalworkers' households with small vernacular translations of the classics (and even Josephus); pharmacists with piles of reading material overflowing shelves and desks; a wine merchant with bags of books in both Italian and, more strikingly, Latin.

The diversity of literary collecting evident in these "extra" cases emerges even more clearly in book owners whose libraries the assessors quantified and that I can accordingly analyze more systematically. The volumes owned by these sixty-seven sub-patrician book owners reveal once again that a taste for literature spanned the major occupational sectors of Venice. These figures also allow us to see some shared tendencies within occupational groups.

BIBLIOPHILIA AND THE URBAN PROFESSIONS

Physicians, eleven of whom appear in these records, outpace all other professions in their book collecting with a median library of 140 volumes. None of these medical men had the resources to build libraries at the level of a Gritti, with his five thousand books, let alone the fifteen-thousand-volume collection of a Cardinal Domenico Grimani.[43] But we should be wary of making a few exceptional patrician libraries the standard for measuring serious collecting. As a group, patricians have often appear desultory literary collectors in historical surveys.[44] Patricians dominate the ranks of consumers studies of art and architecture, but less so in histories of the book. My own findings bear out this general pattern. The range of patrician collections I encountered, while yielding one case of a library that crested two thousand volumes, offer a median of thirty-two volumes, unimpressive given their easy access to educational and literary resources. Indeed, nearly half of the patrician inventories I found that noted the presence of books (thirty-four total) indicated collections of fewer than twenty volumes, and six of these collections involved ten or fewer. By contrast, no inventory for a Venetian physician mentioned fewer than forty-three volumes, and seven of the eleven cases noted more than one hundred volumes. The full range of books physicians collected runs from 43 to 500 volumes, and even the median figure of 140 volumes reveals that Venetian physicians took literary collection seriously.

Second place for passionate book acquisition goes to lawyers (eight individuals), with median collections of 120 books. Close professional kin of lawyers, five secretaries emerge in these records, with a similar median collection of 100 books, with a range of 8 to 261 volumes. Priests, too, make an honorable showing: Twelve men, predominantly parish priests and not the higher clergy, had a median library of ninety-two volumes. Of the men and women directly engaged with the marketplace, pharmacists (six individuals) stand out with a median collection of thirty-four volumes. Few notaries, who occupied a similar place to pharmacists in the professional taxonomy, happened to emerge in these records. But the one notary I did find, Alvise Zorzi, had a library of twenty-nine books, roughly the same size as the collections of our pharmacists.[45] Nine retail merchants also appear, with a median library of twelve volumes, directly comparable to eleven regular artisans whose median collection was eleven volumes.

While these general findings confirm some reasonable suspicions, there are surprises. It makes sense that people associated with the learned professions of law, the chancery, the church, and medicine proved to be book oriented. Families in these circles had clear motive to invest in objects befitting their cultural roles. Similarly, given that families connected to the marketplace had no obvious need to invest extensively in libraries, it also stands to reason that the median collections of merchants and artisans would be smaller than those of lawyers, secretaries, and medical doctors. Yet the fact that retail merchants and artisans still emerge as a significant group of book collectors urges careful thinking about access to and interest in literary material.

Here again it is helpful to return to our secondhand goods dealer, messer Francesco. Even if he could read those Greek manuscripts, he chose to borrow rather than purchase them. Part of his motivation may have been the cachet of association with literati, as I suggested earlier. But it is also unlikely that his budget could have accommodated purchasing such manuscripts; even good print editions of major works, which could run to several ducats if bound, might have proved cost prohibitive. In the negative sense, then, financial limitations surely impacted the reading habits of nonelite families. But in the positive sense, these families may still have been keen readers of diverse material but satisfied their interests through borrowing more than through purchase. As we will see in our case studies, physicians commonly loaned volumes to friends, colleagues, and also to those even less financially and socially solvent than they were. Indeed, an important direction for research in the history of the book would be circulation of texts and borrowing practices outside the ranks of eruditi. For the moment, however, messer Francesco serves as a useful reminder that even when we see relatively small numbers of books in a mercantile or artisanal household, we should not necessarily assume that this indicated less varied material, less readerly passion, or that the individual in question might not have found routes other than ownership to the books they wanted.

The prominence of medical doctors in this inventory evidence also challenges our standard assumption that the clergy and lawyers would have been the more literary-minded professionals—an apparent anomaly that will occupy us centrally in Part II. Beyond the strong showing of physicians, moreover, regular artisans appear with striking regularity. Even if artisans' median collection of eleven books looks modest, it indicates dedicated book buying or preserving, given that the costs of purchase or resistance to obtaining the volumes' resale value would have impacted their domestic budgets more than those of other categories of owners.

In the cases of artisan inventories where assessors provided authors or titles for the volumes, we learn that these owners had rich reading material. Catharina, widow of a goldsmith named Castelino, owned eight books for which the assessors furnished specific information, in addition to "other little ones" that the assessors did not itemize. Catharina's collection filled one cabinet and, according to assessors' estimates, had a total value of two ducats, approximately what her husband had earned per month. Among her devotional literature, we find a vernacular Bible, a breviary, and a meditation on Calvary. In her classical collection appear Lucan (in Italian translation) and the Jewish historian Josephus. Nor did Catharina ignore modern literature; she had copies of Ariosto's *Satires*, the Venetian historian Marcus Antonius Sabellicus's world history, and a collection of contemporary humanist epistles.[46]

These intriguing cases remind us that Benvenuto Cellini was not the only Italian artisan engaged with the humanistic dimensions of Renaissance culture. A goldsmith's widow such as Catharina appears in these laconic references only as a consumer or perhaps even just a conservator of that culture. The books may have belonged to her husband Castelino. Either way, she shows us signs of the Renaissance in an everyday household.

If the books were hers, she strikes a blow at assumptions about readerly interests along the axes of class and gender alike; even if they were her husband's (indeed, even if she herself were illiterate), her decision to conserve these relics of literary culture instead of selling them teaches us, if anything, a more powerful lesson about the perceived value of owning literary objects among the middling ranks of urban society. Put another way, if others working on the scope and reach of humanistic culture such as Brian Maxson point to the entrenchment of humanistic expectations in the daily operations of government, this even more fragmentary evidence suggests those expectations' effects on daily life full stop. Maxson's humanist orations help to explain the dominance of this cultural form by the end of the fifteenth century. But a jeweler's wife harboring copies of Josephus and Ariosto also reminds us that authors cannot exist without readers; literary ideals come into being as much because of their casual subscribers and even excluded aspirants as upon their promulgators.

The practices of pharmacists also reveal vigorous book collecting and occasionally broad literary tastes among the artisanate. Out of six inventories for pharmacists, the median collection was thirty-four volumes, a fairly impressive number. But some pharmacists collected even more assiduously. Adrian Vidal owned sixty volumes.[47] His colleagues Gerolemo a Solimatis and Angilberto Alemani had libraries of 103 and 147 texts, respectively.[48] To judge by the one inventory I encountered from a surgeon, higher artisans within the general field of medicine seem to have had a common tendency to make books priorities. The surgeon Zorzi de Agaziis owned an impressive 239 volumes.[49] Nor were volumes exclusively for occupational use. Solimatis had a penchant for music; half of his collection was in this field. Alemani, German by birth, seems to have been at least bilingual, as only eleven of his books were in German. Although comparatively modest, the collection of Alvisa Bonadia, the widow of a pharmacist, emphasizes once again the range of interests Venetian readers harbored. Bonadia had either acquired or inherited from her husband a good selection of devotional literature, including two offices, a missal, and the epistles of the Evangelists. Nearby, the assessors found Augustine's *Confessions,* Boiardo's *Orlando Innamorato,* and Ariosto's *Orlando Furioso,* as well as two grammar-school primers.[50]

Much as in the case of the goldsmith's widow Catharina, Bonadia's collection shows us an investment in cultural legitimacy. It meant something for Bonadia to own humanistic culture's teaching tools, even if they were her husband's old schoolbooks. Whether used by her children or grandchildren, by herself or by no one at all, owning humanistic textbooks—let alone serious literature ranging from Augustine to Ariosto—marked her home as belonging to the sort of household that valued literary culture and possessed artifacts of that culture.

The inventories of twelve priests, whose social origins were predominantly either artisanal or mercantile, further accentuate the appetite for and value placed on varied literature in Venice's middle ranks. Admittedly, the range of their collections is dramatic: Andrea Marconi owned only five books, whereas Giuseppe Zarlino's library required shelving for 995.[51] As a rule, however, priestly libraries exhibited the same varied tastes as those of our other collectors. Zorzi de Antibaro was atypical in owning mostly theological material: Thirty-eight of his forty books were in his field.[52] More regularly, Venetian priests bought as general readers more than field specialists. Benedetto Premareno, chaplain for the nuns of Santo Sepolcro, had a library estimated to contain twenty-three books plus "others."[53] Of the twenty-three authors or titles provided, only six pertained to Christian theology. His library was better stocked with Seneca, Ovid (both the *Heroides* and the *Fasti*), the epistles of Emperor Claudius, Priscian's genealogy of the gods, Apuleius, Tertullian, Juvenal, Pliny (including an emendation by Ermolao Barbaro), and Josephus. Premareno also had Latin and Greek dictionaries, as well as a few works by contemporary humanists, including the epistles of Sabellico.

The libraries of other priests included large sections of secular literature. Zuanne Argentini was the bishop of Concordia, a position that indicates his higher social status than the other priests we have been discussing. Argentini owned fifty-three books, thirty of which (according to the assessors) were "various works in the humanities."[54] Zuanne Battista Licino, parish priest of San Cassian, had a similar library, despite the fact that his social station was lower than Argentini's. Licino owned fifty-one texts, only nine of which were devotional. The assessors noted that Licino owned twenty folio editions "of various works pertaining to logic and the humanities," as well as twenty-two other volumes about "other things." Licino's humanistic tastes also informed his art collection, which included de rigueur paintings of the Virgin, Mary Magdalene, and Saint Jerome, but extended to portraits of himself, Petrarch and Laura, Virgil, Dante, and the celebrated contemporary poet and salonièrre Vittoria Colonna, marchesa of Pescara.[55] Outpacing his confreres, Antonio Abbardi, the heir of a secondhand goods dealer, had accumulated a 242-volume library. Abbardi's itemized book inventory lists more than 120 classical and contemporary humanist authors, with a special emphasis on ancient Roman comedy.[56]

Much as it is difficult to find a thematic connection between the occupation of selling secondhand goods and the borrowing of Greek philosophical manuscripts, we necessarily puzzle over what parish priests made of their Roman comedies, or how (or even if) a goldsmith's wife read her Josephus and her *Orlando inamorato.* We would have to triangulate inventories with many other sources to arrive at anything like a hypothesis about reading practices, but these inventories tell us one thing for certain: The more categorical we get about who owned what type of books, the more likely we are to misrepresent early-modern readers.

Physicians and lawyers also amassed literary collections that extended far beyond interests or genres relating to their professions. While their predecessors may have focused on occupational and devotional literature, by the sixteenth century urban professionals formed libraries attesting their *scientia* not just their *ars.* We will look at the specific volumes housed in several physicians' libraries in subsequent chapters, but it is worth noting here that medical books in these libraries generally constituted at most a half of the collection, and in most cases a much smaller fraction than that, giving pride of place instead to literature, ancient and modern.[57] Even in cases where it is difficult to determine numbers of volumes in any category, the quality of editions sometimes gives indication of readerly preferences. The 1527 household inventory of Francesco Livello, for instance, noted that he had fewer than twenty books, but among those not worth detailing there lay an office of the Madonna and, next to that, a deluxe edition of Boccaccio.[58] Andrea Benivoli's assessors noted that his 122-volume collection contained only 37 books relating to medicine; the other 85 were of "various" sorts.[59] When we have full book inventories, physicians look even more literary. Medical books make only occasional appearances in the inventory of Alberto Quattrocchi's 339 books and, even counting Aristotle as a medical author, occupational texts formed a scant 4 percent of Alberto Rini's 500-volume library.[60]

Similar to physicians, lawyers collected in a humanistic more than a professional way. If Marcantonio de Noale's professional collection showed a balance between the statutes, legal compendia, and digests necessary for his daily work (44 percent of the 165 volumes) and literary treasures from ancient and modern authors (36 percent), other lawyers reveal their greater appetite for humanistic reading material.[61] Of the 114 texts legible in Ippolito Ganason's 1584 inventory, we see him give 17 percent of his collecting energy to work matters and 83 percent to pleasure—indeed, fully 60 percent of the library comprised ancient and modern literature distinct even from philosophy (4 percent), devotional material (11 percent), natural philosophy or science (4 percent), and general reference (3.75 percent).[62] A kindred spirit, the lawyer Lodovico Usper owned 244 volumes, of which

47 related to the law and 176 did not. Of Usper's 176 literary texts, 120 constituted works drawn from the ancient canon (43 volumes) and modern humanist writing (77 volumes).[63]

These urban professionals might of course have given away the bulk of their professional collections to colleagues or students. If so, that would explain why these posthumous inventories overrepresent literary reading material. Even in that case, however, we would return to the same point by a different route: The humanistic collection constituted their heirs' patrimony. If occupation-specific volumes solidified bonds within the professional community, literary material remained to mark the family's humanistic cultural credibility.

What about retail merchants? As with artisans, merchants' median collection of twelve volumes seems slim. Yet the range was wide in this case, too: from six to 105 volumes. And when we get any description of the books, we once again find great variety. A wool merchant called Zampiero de Alessandri displayed in his great room a collection of saints' lives and an office of the Madonna, together with Ariosto, Petrarch, and Giovanni Boccaccio's *On Famous Women (Delle donne illustri),* most likely the revised and amplified version of this encyclopedia of female achievement that had recently been published by the humanist and *poligrafo* Giuseppe Betussi.[64] Florio Audet, a Cypriot trader, had a more extensive library of fifty-nine volumes, two of which were written in Greek, and the rest were noted as books "for studying."[65] Another wool merchant, Paolo son of Agustin, amassed fifty-eight "printed books of various kinds."[66] Even at the lower end of the mercantile bracket, we still find literature. An innkeeper, Giacomo de Pergo, owned "ten printed books" that the assessors did not itemize; they did make note, however, of Pergo's deluxe edition of Dante.[67]

The diversity of these sixteenth-century Venetian book owners reveals both continuity and change in the city's history of literary consumption. Susan Connell found similar categories of book owners for the years 1345–1480.[68] Connell's collectors included merchants, lawyers, priests, one doctor, and an engraver, very similar to the categories of owner I find regularly appearing for the period 1500–1630. So, too, Cecchini and Zorzi found *cittadini* appearing more regularly than patricians as owners of books, even if their collections tended to be smaller.

Yet the collectors we have been meeting here suggest some different patterns. The one physician that Connell found, Pietro Tomasi, was the only individual in her group to have accumulated more than 40 volumes; he owned 130 books.[69] Zorzi also noted a few cases of physicians with remarkable book collections, including a professor of medicine at Padua, Guilandino di Mareinburgo, whose 1589 bequest increased the Marciana's holdings in printed books by nearly two thousand volumes.[70] Inasmuch we see physicians exhibiting acute bibliomania, these medical doctors have much in common with my own cases. Yet Tomasi's singularity as a physician-humanist marks a distinction between these earlier centuries and the era of our protagonists. Members of the medical profession are so much more numerous in sixteenth-century records than they are in fifteenth—a distinction that Zorzi's data might also have borne out, but he did not tabulate ownership according to profession across his total sample.

What Zorzi's data and my own certainly bear out, however, is the diminution in the relative presence of patricians between Connell's early Renaissance cases and our late Renaissance cases. Patricians comprised 30 percent of Connell's total group of book owners, whereas Zorzi found patricians in only 5 percent of inventories that included books; in my larger group of inventories, patricians only comprise 34 percent of book owners. And both Zorzi and I find that, on average, the number of volumes patricians owned paled in comparison to citizens. While some patrician families built vast libraries, most patricians had roughly the same number of books in their homes as artisans did and, in some cases, fewer.

Yet important differences also emerge between even Zorzi's cases and mine with regard to the numerical representation of artisans. If it is not surprising that, considering the last decades of manuscript and the first of print, Connell found only one artisan book owner, it is striking that Zorzi's sample yielded only 5 percent cases of artisans. By contrast, artisans comprise 19 percent of my group.

Another more general shift emerges in this comparison: Sixteenth-century collectors as a group were more numerous and their libraries much larger than their fourteenth- and fifteenth-century predecessors. While all but one of Connell's collectors owned fewer than forty volumes, my 101 collectors (comprising all categories) owned on average eighty-five volumes.[71] In part, these dramatic spikes reflect the relative affordability of books in the sixteenth century. Even granted that books were more affordable in the sixteenth century, however, one still needed to learn how to read. Thus we should keep in mind that access to education also played an essential role in Venetian intellectual life.

It may be useful at this point to look more closely at what we know about Venetian literacy, especially in the late sixteenth century. Drawing on an unusually helpful set of "professions of faith" that the Venetian government required of all teachers in independent, communal, and church schools in 1587–1588, Paul Grendler has revealed a pedagogical workforce of 245 instructors that he estimates served 26 percent of the city's school-age boys (and .2 percent of school-age girls).[72] Grendler also notes, however, that these figures must constitute a minimum, given several other possible avenues for the acquisition of literacy. Venice's wealthier citizens would often have hired private tutors for their children. It was also fairly common for those with some means to send their daughters to convents as "boarders," which not only kept the girls away from sexual danger in the years before marriage but often provided substantive instruction as well. He further observes that parents might also have taught their children at home, estimating that another 1 percent of the population learned in this way. There were, moreover, catechism schools that met on Sundays and holidays, which offered intermittent instruction in morals, reading, and writing. All things considered, then, Grendler suggests that roughly 33 percent of Venetian boys and 12–13 percent of girls would have achieved literacy through one or another of these means.[73] There are logical grounds for seeing this estimate as a very bare minimum. The "professions of faith" on which Grendler's figures most rely offer a useful snapshot, but these sources (like all sources) are also problematic. At least a few instructors would have left the city for some reason in the years before the profession was required, and others may have found ways to fly under the radar in the years following. Moreover, there is no telling how many thousands of students made their way through the catechism schools. And "homeschooling" must have affected more than Grendler's meager (and unexplained) estimate of 1 percent of the population. Even if only 26 percent of men and women had access to a full grammar-school education, it is hard to believe that they would so seldom have made their children beneficiaries of their own instruction. In this sense, it seems best to keep in mind the far more optimistic figures that Robert Black has offered.[74] Even if we would not want to propose literacy rates of 60 percent in an Italian urban center, we are surely safer in thinking of at least 40 percent given all the likely avenues of education.

What are we even looking for when we set out to examine "literacy"? Armando Petrucci has gone furthest in pluralizing our too-often unitary conception of interactions with the written word to describe the range of possibilities evident in the premodern world, from reading and writing fluently in multiple languages to forms of "semiliteracy" in the vernacular, as well as visual and pictorial literacies.[75] Petrucci stopped with the Trecento, but the possibilities he located continued to operate centuries later and, in the case of skills in vernacular reading and writing, to expand with each generation.

In short, by the sixteenth century a solid education was within reach for men and women of the artisanal and mercantile classes. Venetians' collecting practices underscore a generalized desire to invest in education and books. These trends are attributable not just to costs and availability of schools and books but also to the more nebulous, but nonetheless perceptible, entrenchment of humanistic ideals.[76] The increasing cachet attached to the literary may also have inspired a diversification of readerly palates. As Connell showed, book owners of the early Renaissance tended to acquire volumes in two categories: professional or practical texts and manuals, together with the most widely read literature of the day, especially Cicero and Dante. Zorzi revealed more diverse tastes, suggesting a fourfold typology of libraries that did not necessarily break down according to the owner's status: books for spiritual, professional, or day-to-day necessities; books for cultivated people who were not literati or scholars; books for humanists and scholars; and "princely" libraries collected by the wealthy (and most often but not always patrician) families to make available to others as a form of patronage.[77] The collections we have explored here, and will continue to consider in subsequent chapters, reveal similarly broad interests encompassing different social groups. We need think only of Catharina, the goldsmith's wife, whose small library included the Roman poet Lucan and the historian Josephus.

READING PUBLICS IN VENICE AND EUROPE

Were the boundaries of cultural possibility exceptionally broad in the Republic of Venice? To be sure, Venice was in certain respects sui generis. A fulcrum for the book trade, La Serenissima also housed perhaps Europe's most apathetic branch of the Holy Office.[78] On the other hand, urban centers in general offered ready access to education and to diverse reading material. Teachers headed for cities, as court appointments were in short supply and difficult to secure in a pedagogical marketplace flooded with underemployed humanists. We recall that Grendler found 245 professed schoolteachers as of 1587–1588, an impressive number for an urban center roughly the size of Manhattan's Central Park. Similarly, most printers set up shop in cities to secure the widest possible market for their wares.

Venice's literary consumption, while perhaps more voracious than elsewhere, still had much in common with other urban centers in Italy and in Europe. Christian Bec, for instance, surveyed Florentine library inventories of the fifteenth and sixteenth century and unearthed hundreds of "middling sort" book collectors.[79] As early as the first half of the fifteenth century, forty out of fifty-two Florentine book owners whose profession could be determined belonged to the mercantile bracket of society.[80]

Sixteenth-century Venetian mercantile and artisanal book owners also had a great deal in common with seventeenth-century Romans of the same social sectors, to judge by Renata Ago's findings.[81] Among her paradigmatic cases are two lawyers of the Negrelli and Pari families and a patrician-lawyer of the Neruzzi clan, who each owned more than four hundred volumes. Equally impressive are her artisanal protagonists, including a painter with a collection of 160 volumes, a goldsmith with 97, and an embroiderer with 58. Much as we have seen in the case of Venetians, moreover, Roman artisans tended to equal or trump mercantile collectors. Among her merchant subjects, one (a banker) amassed forty-nine books; the other two had only ten volumes each. And, as with our Venetian book owners, Ago has found that Romans bought widely. Her three central cases of sub-patrician bibliophiles, a lawyer of the Pari family, a goldsmith of the Cangiani family, and a painter of the Raspantini family, show us libraries that gave due space to religious material (between 10 and 28 percent of their owners' total collections) but abounded in the humanities, especially literature, history, and the arts.[82]

The sketch of the Venetian book-owning public that I have offered here also meshes with Albert Labarre's collectors in sixteenth-century Amiens, drawn from his own wide survey of household inventories.[83] Of Labarre's 4,442 inventories, only 887 (20 percent) listed books of any type. Although I examined only 1,227 inventories, the percentage of those that mention books is similar (18 percent)—perhaps even more similar in the final analysis, since I screened out all inventories in which only one book was listed, whereas he included owners of a single volume. Of Labarre's inventories, 703 indicated occupation or status, and in this subgroup he found a similar range of noble, clerical, medical, mercantile, and artisanal owners. Considering professions by group, the rates of book ownership in Amiens were highest for the same subsectors of the population that we have found here: physicians (94 percent), lawyers (73 percent), and priests (72 percent). So, too, the nobility of Amiens, while high in rates of book ownership (70 percent), tended, like Venetian patricians, to have comparatively small libraries.

Two differences emerge between Labarre's survey and mine, however, and these differences parallel those between Connell's findings for the fifteenth century and my own for the later Renaissance. First, like Connell, Labarre found relatively few physicians; they were serious collectors, but comprised only 18 cases out of his 703 book owners (2 percent). Sixteenth-century Venetian physicians, by contrast, held their own in the ranks of "book people," constituting 18 of the 101 collectors who emerged in my inventories. Second, Labarre's book owners, like Connell's, tended to form professional libraries. By contrast, sixteenth-century Venetian book owners collected broadly.

Venetian literary consumers thus urge us to revise some common claims in the history of the book, especially the notion that (even in the sixteenth century) readers seldom owned more than a Bible or collections of saints' lives.[84] While this may be statistically accurate for large geopolitical regions and certainly for Europe as a whole, urban localities often tell a different story. We have not only seen members of the learned professions purchasing across genres; we have also seen merchants and even artisans who had comparatively few volumes lying around but those volumes were as likely to be Dante, or even Josephus, as they were to be devotional material. Given the omnivorous collections of physicians, moreover, we should also rethink our assumption that members of the professions formed primarily "professional" libraries. As we see in more detail hereafter, physicians' libraries tilted toward literature and away from medical texts, and even the works of moral philosophy within their occupational remit. Collectively, Venetian literary consumers tell us that books in the humanities had become a priority for diverse buyers working with divergent financial constraints and levels of education.

LITERATURE AND DAILY LIFE: A WAY FORWARD

Inventories have shown us that a Hellenophilic retailer, rather than being an anomaly, had much in common with Venice's reading public, characterized as it was by a surprising range of actors and literary tastes. But how much did Venetians' reading mesh with other aspects of their lives? Or, put a different way, how else might everyday people have showed their interest in literature?

One possible route for deepening our sense of literature's impact on lives of the middle ranks lies not in inventories but in other family documents, and not tracking books as such but the names of authors and characters in Venetians' naming practices. Names drawn from the classical and humanistic canon have emerged already among the book owners we have encountered and indeed of the many others whom I could not incorporate into the analysis. I am not claiming that all those who named their sons Marc'Antonio or their daughters Polissena consciously invoked ancient Roman statesmen or Homeric heroines; they might simply have wished to give their children the same names as well-known contemporaries. Yet classical naming did make a statement. We know that the names of saints and deceased relatives, which in most cases amounted to the same thing, provided the common stock of children's names.[85] Outliers, then, endowed their children with a form of cultural legitimacy.

The classical tradition offered a lineage as venerable as the Christian tradition—and in fact a "classier" one, from a worldly point of view. Prescriptive treatises did not specify what names were appropriate for a given social rank, but we can see evidence that pagan names were used to gain or signal cachet in Venetian convent records. It seems that nuns had long used the moment of pronouncing vows as an opportunity to upgrade ordinary given names derived from the usual catalogue of saints and martyrs to more striking professed names drawn from antiquity. Concerned about this practice, the Patriarch of Venice in 1692 penned a detailed memorandum concerning the novitiate, in which he reminded the convent that novices must not choose pagan names in the course of their professions, but instead take the names of Catholic saints.[86]

Not all testators explained why they chose a particular name for their children, but instances of disclosure articulate the desire to provide heirs, especially those who were socially disadvantaged, with a form of cosmetic honor. One self-described citizen named Placido Ragazzoni had an illegitimate son whom he recognized in his will of 1570 and hoped to legitimize in the fullest sense of that term. Ragazzoni's family had no history of unusual names, but he called his son Scipione, noting, "[Scipione] was first baptized with the name Beneto [the name of Ragazzoni's father], but later, regretting that our father's name should be passed down to an illegitimate child, I renamed him Scipione, and so he continues to be called."[87] After giving the boy the name of an illustrious ancient Roman, this father then turned to the topic of educational social mobility, insisting, "About this boy: it has been and remains my wish that he apply himself to the liberal arts, and thereby make a man of himself."[88] In Ragazzoni's view, his son's name and his success in literary studies were mutually reinforcing social assets. At the very least, by naming his son Scipione, Ragazzoni underscored his own familiarity with Roman literature and history.

Considering all the families who hinted at their reading habits in their naming practices would require a book of its own. But it is worth sketching my initial findings here, as they underscore the literary convictions of middle-rank Venetians. Above all, I hope that this glance at naming practices across an urban population might inspire further research in this vein.

Classical naming appears with notable regularity among physicians and medical practitioners, the group we have already seen and will continue to see especially eager to prove their cultural legitimacy. Instead of traditional Venetian names, the physician Francesco Longo gave three of his four children Roman names: Giulio, Cornelio, Virginia.[89] A number of Longo's medical colleagues similarly took the classical route in naming their children. Valerio Superchio named his three sons after two emperors and a Virgilian hero (Tiberio, Alessandro, and Ascanio) and Benedetto Rini called two of his sons Fabrizio and Scipione.[90] We learn from Scipione Rini's will that one of his nephews was called Marco Aurelio.[91] Another physician, Agostino Tomasini, had bountiful progeny that included a Camilla, a Lucrezia, an Alessandro, and a Prospero.[92] A physician of the Monaldi family, himself named Ottavian, gave his illegitimate son the name Camillo.[93] Pharmacists, too, regularly took the classical turn. An apothecary of the Copazzo family, himself named Orfeo, called his daughter Virginia.[94] Another, called Pietro, named his eldest son Zuanne (John), but gave his younger sons the names Scipione and Prospero.[95] Still another pharmacist, Ludovico Usper, named one of his daughters Faustina; this Faustina married a physician named Aurelio.[96] Another of Usper's daughters, Anzelica, also married a physician, Andrea Baranzon of Modena. In Anzelica Baranzon's will, written in her own hand (as she proudly stated four times in the course of the document), she adopted a certain Cesare, Baranzon's son from a previous marriage, as her own child and heir.[97] Most striking are the choices made by Adrian (Hadrian) Vidal, a pharmacist, who named his children Laelio, Letizia, Diodoro, Eugenio, and Plinio.[98]

The classical naming trend also emerges, if more sporadically, among wine merchants, architects, barber-surgeons, grammar-school teachers, booksellers, and painters. We even find the occasional tile worker, coppersmith, rope winder, carver, dyer, stonecutter, or street cleaner sporting or bestowing ancient Greek and Roman names. Cornelia, the daughter of a barber, had married a coppersmith named Alessandro; her sister was named Lucrezia; and her will was witnessed by a secondhand goods dealer named Marcantonio.[99] Admittedly, these individual appearances of classical names might have had any number of inspirations, especially as we move into the sectors of society in which we tend to find relatively few book owners. But when classical names start grouping, we have more reason to suspect that the family in question had some familiarity with literature. Consider, for instance, a carver named Francesco, whose sister was named Camilla, and who gave his daughter the name of Daria, who in turn named her son Orazio.[100] A street cleaner called Matteo named his sons Camillo and Virgilio, and one of these sons named his own daughter Vittoria.[101] One family of stonecutters had a father named Tullius and a son named Marc'Antonio; another stonecutter named his daughter Polissena.[102]

Classical and humanistic naming practices emerge with sufficient frequency that we can hope to find a substantial number of potential case studies, but at the same time they are unusual enough, especially among families of sub-patrician rank, to suggest considered strategy. When classical names do emerge in a family, it would be worth looking for other signs of reading within their kin group. Consider for a moment the case of the pharmacist Adrian Vidal. The name Adrian (Hadrian) itself catches the eye. Families drew some names regularly from the ancient record, including Helena, Marcantonio, Lucrezia, Alessandro, even Scipione. The name Hadrian seldom emerges. Accordingly, if we were encountering him for the first time, we might do well to see if the family records turn up anything more relating to books or education. In this case, such an effort yields positive results. Adrian Vidal took a highly creative approach in naming his children. If the physician Valerio Superchio showed some literary flair in naming his sons after two emperors and a well-known figure of mythology, Vidal's naming a son after Diodorus Siculus showed still more. Shifting back to the world of inventories, then, we find that this creative parent also owned a substantial amount of reading material. Vidal's library included sixty volumes, according to assessors. Going further into the archives, we also discover that he had seen to the advanced education of his daughter as well as his sons. In an age in which a distinct minority of testators wrote their own wills, women formed a tiny fraction of that minority. Yet Letizia Vidal's own testament exists in autograph.[103]

A classical fashion in naming, then, encompassed much of Venetian society. And fashions, by nature, relate to status. To be sure, not every Venetian stonecutter read Cicero, but Venetian stonecutters who named their sons Marcantonio instead of Zuanne were making a status claim; they may have done so by direct reference to antiquity or by reference to the names chosen by patricians. And we know patricians to have routinely embellished their own family honor by tethering themselves to the classical tradition—sometimes literally, in cases of imaginative genealogies dating back to antiquity. A more extensive examination of classicizing naming practices might give us indications of a variety of families that affiliated themselves with humanistic currents. Classical naming might be another means to track the diffusion of literary culture.

At all events, the Venetian reading public we have met in this chapter urges eschewing a paradigm of "elite" versus "popular" culture. As messer Francesco the manuscript-hunting retailer suggested through his singular example and as we have now seen in inventories at large, Renaissances took place across the middle ranks of Venetian society. Where we might have expected to find, in general, professionals with books useful for their day jobs, and most everyone else with devotional material and tales of marvels, we have instead found idiosyncratic assortments of reading material across social groups. Evidence of commerce with the humanities, if not always with the classics, pops up on the shelves, tables, and sometimes in the genealogies of university-trained men, merchants, parish priests, and wives of artisans.

Owning books and perhaps naming children after the figures encountered there signified an investment in literary culture. As useful as they are in helping us find people who made those cultural investments, however, inventories only hint at motivations and priorities—and tell us less still about literary practices. In search of more direct testimony of the literary and social ideals encouraging Venice's readers, we turn now to their final wills.

CHAPTER 2

TESTAMENTARY HUMANISM

Venetians from all social sectors wrote wills. Among the city's artisanal, mercantile, and professional sectors, however, individuals tended to leave testaments that evinced a preoccupation with literary and pedagogical matters. The concern about cultural legitimacy we find in testaments offers us a more detailed view of this ideal and its motivations than we could draw from inventories. Given the constraints within which testaments were produced—old age, ill health, physical danger, limited budgets for enlisting notarial services, and above all the notary's mandate to optimize the legal clarity and relevance of their clients' remarks—even brief discursive departures had deep significance. Stanley Chojnacki and many others in recent years have taught us to read wills not only to find connections but to understand relationships, gender dynamics, family strategies, and the nuances of emotional bonds.[1] Inspired by this work and the outstanding research on Hebrew "ethical wills," I read Venetian wills for the literary.[2]

On the basis of that reading, I classify as practitioners of what I am calling "testamentary humanism" not only the rare cases of testators who made direct literary references but also testators who mentioned their own literary or pedagogical endeavors, specified book bequests, allocated particular sums for the education of kin, or exhorted relatives to improve themselves through study. I also classify as testamentary humanists those who departed most dramatically from the notarial boilerplate in giving miniature lectures on ethics that foregrounded *virtù* in ways that may have been compatible with Christian morality but that leaned harder on classical definitions of *virtus* as fortitude, industry, and accomplishment.

Testamentary humanists did not follow an established practice of making a will particular to literati. There was no such "best practice," even if, as Christopher Celenza has shown, a few humanists such as Petrarch, Niccolò Niccoli, and Giannozzo Manetti did bequeath (or at least planned to bequeath) their libraries to their communities.[3] Disposing of a book collection in this way enhanced the scholar's reputational afterlife but, as Celenza shows, contemporary society had also come to expect that scholars would establish libraries for public use.[4] Even if we can find a tradition of humanists bequeathing books, however, we find no special forms of testamentary discourse among them. By "testamentary humanism," then, I mean to indicate the desire of an individual to explore more fully the discursive potential of the testament as a document, a desire we find most among the people who did not have the access to literary expression that humanists enjoyed. Practitioners of testamentary humanism went out of their way to disclose the Renaissances writ small taking place in their houses, sometimes because the testament was their primary or even their only way to record that efflorescence.

Book bequests and references to education represent the form of testamentary humanism that most closely resembles the evidence of book ownership we have just considered. But unlike numbers with scant descriptions, the books that appear in testaments are fortunately situated in a document that gives us at least a few more clues as to the owner's social and cultural place, as well as their priorities. Accordingly, we will begin with general references to books in Venetians' wills, turning thereafter to more discursive material such as mention of particular texts or titles and, above all, the claims to cultural legitimacy inspiring the ethical precepts on which some testators lectured their beneficiaries.

Venetian practitioners of testamentary humanism will occasionally recall the enigmatic messer Francesco the retailer to us. These men and women, like him and like the majority of the Venetian book collectors we have met, belonged to society's middle ranks. Once again, while no laborers emerge, precious few patricians did either. The types of people who made books, learning, and ethical bequests priorities in their testaments continue to be those who occupied the dynamic social spaces between the decidedly underserved and the robustly enfranchised. While we cannot with any certainty posit the motives inspiring messer Francesco to seek Greek manuscripts, many of our testamentary humanists explain in their wills exactly what their books meant to them and what they hoped beneficiaries would do to preserve the volumes and to enhance the family's cultural assets. The search for honor served as an engine for literary, educational, and ethical endeavor. In short, cultural legitimacy emerges here, too, as both a practical and an idealistic aim.

BEQUEATHING BOOKS AND EDUCATION

Federico Leon, a parish priest of San Jacopo in the district of Rialto, divided his library among several categories of people.[5] Leon left his books of theology in Latin, Greek, and Hebrew to a local chapter of Capuchin friars, because they were "scholars of the humanities and Christian doctrine alike." His Bible and three-volume collection of the theologian Nicholas of Lyra went to his colleague and friend, Father Bernardin Polo. Leon left a deluxe manuscript edition of the Psalms to Giovanni Battista Contarini, his "most honored patron," a member of one of Venice's ducal families, and to Contarini's sons, whom he had tutored. Leon asked that Contarini accept and protect this copy of the Psalms, because they were especially valuable: "they have been translated verbatim by Master Elias the Jew. I wrote them down as he dictated them to me." Leon allows that some of his fellow priests might also consult this precious manuscript, but he reminds them to take care, as "they are written in my own hand legibly and are the translation of Master Elias the Jew who was once my teacher, a most learned man in the Holy Tongue—and I wrote them down verbatim, with great diligence." Although only a parish priest, Leon shared the humanist celebrity Isaac Casaubon's passion for acquiring "authentic" Hebrew learning from Jewish intellectuals, a desire recently and eloquently explicated by Anthony Grafton and Joanna Weinberg.[6] Leon's investment in literary culture also had classical dimensions. His library was stocked with humanistic material. "All my books of the humanities," he explains, "whether small or large, should go to my nephews who are studying good and ethical literature." In making this bequest, Leon left on record his own commitment to humanistic pursuits while at the same time pointing out the intellectual attainments of his family members and his wish to support them in these worthy endeavors. In so doing, this parish priest proved his cultural legitimacy and, transmitting it to his nephews through his gift, urged them to take his honorable legacy further.

Not all clergy were as detailed as Leon in commenting on their cultural passions, but many seem to have shared his priorities. A man who described himself as Francesco, chaplain and confessor at the convent of Sant'Alvise, made his brother, a secondhand goods dealer, his principal beneficiary. But Francesco did make particular mention of his books, which he bequeathed to one of his students.[7] Father Luca de Zorzi left his Bible to a colleague, together with the works of the medieval French theologian Jean Gerson and one other work of theology. He bequeathed the remainder of his books to a young man named Zuanne, whom he characterizes as the son of one of his maids but who might also have been his own illegitimate son.[8] Father Giovanni Solerio, like Father Leon, favored his nephews, bequeathing to his brother's sons all of his books "except the canonical texts printed here in Venice," which he gave to his confessor.[9]

Among priests, who at least theoretically did not have children, book bequests often signaled bonds of extended kinship. But the transmission of texts also reinforced friendships. Thomaso Fontana gave "three pairs of books, whichever he likes" to his friend, a merchant named Francesco Bon.[10] Zorzi di Michiel bequeathed all his books to the nephew of a widow named Lodovica, in recognition for her care during his illness; this bequest, unlike the money he left to his natural daughter, niece, and others, honored his caretaker for her service in a way that represented her family as the sort of people who appreciated the more abstract valuables to be found in words on pages.[11]

Bibliographic bequests also emerge in the wills of laymen who, like priests, found themselves without legitimate bodily heirs. A French merchant named Symone Flossigliera, for instance, left as his universal beneficiary a nephew whom, he says, "both I myself and my wife have taken as our own son."[12] The estate of which this nephew was the beneficiary included Flossigliera's "books, arms, and clothes." Whether clerical or lay, testators could use book bequests to showcase their intellectual honor, which in turn redounded to their family and friends. For people whose social station or profession were not automatically associated with high literary endeavors, true both for the parish priests and for the retail merchants we have been meeting, the possession of books had a peculiar significance. The more humble or problematic the testator's social station, the more they had (and sought) to prove in cultural terms.

The social significance of literary possessions emerges with a particular clarity when we consider those testaments in which books are absent or marginal concerns. Literary bequests, always rare, become even more so in patrician wills. The urban nobility evidently did not feel the need to construct their "virtue" in the same way as Venetians of the middle ranks. Camillo Donà, writing his will in 1593, noted his extensive library; but he seemed content that his mother and heir would sell it after his death. Donà only urged her to get the best possible price for his Greek manuscripts, as he had troubled to transcribe them himself.[13] Vettor Marcello did not discuss any books of his own; rather, he mentions texts only in passing, noting that his son Marcantonio had purchased "with his own money, earned from his own activities" certain books, furniture, antiquities, and tapestries, which Marcantonio should not be forced to divide with his brothers.[14] While there were no doubt ardently humanistic Venetian patricians (we need only think of Pietro Bembo), none such emerged in the wills I examined. The patricians whose testaments I encountered seem to have taken their abundant social and often financial capital as sufficient markers of their quality, displaying little concern with their cultural capital.[15]

Books emerge as a priority for those outside the ranks of patricians, but education brings us an even more diverse group of people and further indications of the connections between intellectual engagement, social anxiety, and cultural legitimacy at society's middle. If we might have doubted that a retailer possessed sufficient education to read Greek philosophy or even have heard of it, testators of the middle ranks suggest that our doubts might have been misguided. The desire to encourage, or pressure, young relatives into substantive and even university educations percolated in precisely messer Francesco's social sector. Men and women of the middle ranks seem to have been especially keen that their children prove themselves to be "of the right sort" by means of education.

The testators most obsessed with education came from the world of medicine, but other categories of people in that swath of society between laborers and patricians also made a strong showing. Physicians and their wives represent eleven of the twenty-six testators who were either insistent on the education of their relatives or else determined to display their own learning. But we also find here three retail merchants and a self-described "citizen" who probably also belonged to the world of the marketplace, as well as two priests, two lawyers, one lawyer's wife, a pharmacist's wife, a barber-surgeon, and a glassblower. By contrast, only three patrician wills mentioned education, and, as we will see, patricians' remarks reveal a very different attitude toward that desideratum.

In several cases, testators who bequeathed books also emphasized education. One such case is the parish priest, Father Leon, whom we met earlier. Not only was this cleric proud of his authoritative translation of the Psalms and a supporter of his nephew's education, he also offered a brief account of his career as an educator. His patron, Giovanni Battista Contarini, had hired Leon to tutor his children. Accordingly, Leon had lived for a number of years in Contarini's principal residence, where he enjoyed free room and board, as well as an annual stipend of twenty-five ducats. Leon left his post two years before his agreement with Contarini had expired, however, and Leon specified in his will that his executors must repay the five hundred ducats that he considered Contarini to be owed for two years' worth of stipends, room, and board.

Another parish priest, Paulo Pincio, followed Leon in making a point of his intellectual labors. Pincio, however, was more emphatic and self-referential. "I am fifty-seven years old," Pincio begins. "My spirit sags from fretting over the many and burdensome worries that always accompany our lives, just as my body is worn out from the continual vigils and efforts of my studies."[16] Like others whom we have encountered and others whom we will meet hereafter, Pincio seized the narrative potential of the testament to sketch, however briefly, the self-portrait of a scholar.

If few testators expatiated on their studies as much as Pincio, their wills more commonly make bequests to teachers that honored their past service and put the families' own investment in education on record. Helena Usper, wife of the lawyer and musical impresario Lodovico Usper, left her son's tutor a bequest of cash.[17] We might perhaps dismiss Signora Usper's generosity as noblesse oblige, given that she was the wife of a man prominent in her city's cultural life. Yet very different categories of people made similar bequests. For instance, Laura Codega, the daughter of a printer and wife of a perfumer, marked her family's participation in the world of learning through small cash bequests to a Donna Caterina who had tutored her and her sister.[18] From one point of view, Helena Usper and Laura Codega both had more pressing matters to attend to in their testaments than remembering the labors of a tutor. From a Christian perspective, the primary objective of the testament was the disposition of the soul, making this document a component of salvation, as Samuel Cohn's work on pious expressions and bequests in Sienese testaments has shown us.[19] Making room for matters that were inessential spiritually and even legally (neither Usper nor Codega needed to reimburse their tutors), both women suggest the deep meaning that education held for them. Coming from such different social spaces, moreover, these two testators reinforce for us that valuation of the life of the mind crossed social categories—and gender categories. If Usper inhabits a more traditional role of matriarch supporting her son's education, Codega suggests the pride that a woman of artisan rank took in the fact that she had received tutoring.

The stakes of education rose when testators had illegitimate or otherwise disadvantaged heirs whose social position they hoped to secure or improve. The priest Paolo Pincio had one such heir, his son Felippo. Felippo labored under a triple stigma: he was illegitimate, the son of a priest, and, worse still, his father's place in the ecclesiastical hierarchy was almost literally nowhere. It was difficult enough for a Pietro Bembo, a wealthy

Venetian patrician and a cardinal, not only to ensure his intellectual legacy in textual terms but also to place his well-educated but still illegitimate children in society.[20] Imagine the situation for Pincio, the parish priest of Muggia, a harbor town covering a grand total of five square miles in the southeast region of Trieste on the border of modern-day Slovenia. Pincio had a difficult task before him in protecting and promoting Felippo.

The first component of Pincio's strategy for advancing his heir was to put the best possible gloss on his son's arrival in the world. Far from branding Felippo as an accident, less still as the unfortunate result of desire getting the better of his vow of celibacy, he celebrates his heir with refreshing verve. Pincio terms Felippo his "dearest and sweetest little son," explaining, "[He is] the child that I had with Donna Crestina, a woman with excellent manners and habits, in the last phase of my life and more to ensure that my family would have some successor (which is a natural desire) than to satisfy any voluptuous appetite."[21] This discursive display was the best means at Pincio's disposal for legitimizing his son. The proceeds of his miniscule benefice could not furnish the cash necessary to buy a dispensation. Yet he could acknowledge Felippo, represent Filippo's mother as a fine woman with excellent manners, and compliment himself on having furnished his dwindling patriline with an heir.

Pincio also did everything possible to ensure that Felippo would receive a substantive education, which he viewed as the linchpin of his son's future reputation. Assisting Pincio in this pedagogical strategy were two friends, Alessandro Ziliol and Galeazzo Macio, both lawyers who held joint doctorates in civil and canon law. Pincio begs Ziliol and Macio, who are also his executors, to look on Felippo as their own son and "to the extent that they can, see to it that he is raised in the fear of God and that he keeps studying." Underscoring the critical place of academic attainments for Felippo's future, Pincio addresses his son in an urgent hortatory register in the final paragraph of his will. "Attend to your studies," he commands, "bearing in mind that it falls to you to maintain the honor of this family. You are the last of us. And from my study, which I leave to you as a memento of my vigils, you will come to know how I have acquired everything of which you are now the heir. I never had anything from my father or my mother except my birth." If Felippo studies, his father concludes, "you will earn honor and profit and, in the end, you will be dear to God and to men."[22] For Pincio, education was an essential component of honor and a prerequisite for social advancement—perhaps always the case, but especially so for a young man with a social stigma to surmount.

Nicolò Paruta, a lawyer, also had an illegitimate son, Zuan Andrea, whom he legitimized through his will and made his universal heir. Paruta bestowed on Zuan Andrea a fulsome paternal benediction akin to Pincio's and reminded Zuan Andrea that if he wishes to "be taken for an honorable man," he must go to university. "I want him to study law," Paruta instructs his executors, "given that (so far as I can tell) he is hardworking and intelligent."[23] A self-described "citizen" named Placido Ragazzoni also had an illegitimate son and heir, Scipione, on whose education hinged his future reputation. "I want him to attend to literary studies," Ragazzoni commented to his executors. "It is by this means that he may become a man."[24] The gender rhetoric typically encountered in early-modern texts has accustomed scholars to construing masculinity as constituted by dominance in political, martial, and above all sexual contexts.[25] Queer theory and lines of inquiry concerning male friendship have helped tremendously in nuancing our conceptions of early-modern masculinities, but here too we have a distance to go still in incorporating those new approaches into our interpretive frameworks.[26] Questions about academic or intellectual masculinity, among many, clearly repay examination.[27] As ever, we can pursue answers not only in published texts, journals, correspondence, and contemporary drama but also in archival records. Placido Ragazzoni states plainly if laconically that literary studies will confer honorable manhood on his illegitimate son. The securest explanation for what Ragazzoni meant is that literary studies, things of inherent rather than worldly value, could offer Scipione cultural legitimacy that might compensate for biological illegitimacy—much the same confident hope Father Leon expressed for his own illegitimate son. But within this more general meaning lurks a statement about gender paradigms as well. Ragazzoni conceived of "making yourself a man" not as performing dominance in any simple way but instead as earning respect, or counting for something. With this intriguing definition of manhood in mind, we can see how literary studies, given their high social no less than intellectual valuation, would offer an efficient route to masculine honor specifically, no less than to cultural legitimacy more generally.

Even parents with legitimate children spoke of the social power of education in the same terms. A wine merchant called Zuanne Farsina asked his executors to ensure that his son pursue the life of the mind "so that he may become a man of the right sort."[28] Offering us an expression a bit more specific than Ragazzoni's, Farsina envisioned his heir not only becoming a man but becoming a *uomo da bene*. One might translate this phrase as "an honest man," "a good man," or "a man of the right sort." Farsina did not encourage his executors to see to it that his son went to church and confession to become "a good man." Nor, for that matter, did he specify training that would encourage his son to become an honest businessman. Instead, Farsina saw book learning as the route to virtue, ethics, and quality. This wine merchant may or may not have been a reader of humanist writing, but he had imbibed two central claims to be found there: Education built character, and an outstanding one promised exceptional ethics and accomplishments. Farsina vests his most ardent hopes for cultural legitimacy in his son, which might suggest that he had not enjoyed access to the studies he wanted his son to undertake. This merchant insisted that his son receive an education that did not directly connect the boy to his father's occupation, as would have seemed the more obvious family strategy, but instead might take him in new directions. Whatever the young man did to earn a living, Farsina envisioned a serious education ensuring his son's reputation, a vision shared with so many others we have encountered. If he followed his father's injunctions, the junior Farsina might indeed have become another messer Francesco, that is, a merchant well acquainted with texts for reading and at least tangentially connected to the humanistic communities forming around them.

EDUCATION IN WHAT—AND FOR WHAT?

Venetian testators often spoke of education and "letters," but we should pause and consider what particular skills or studies they had in mind. If these middling-sort testators did not all imagine their children reading philosophical manuscripts in ancient Greek (though some may have done), we can be certain that when they spoke of education, they had substantive studies in mind. Ronald Witt, Paul Grendler, Robert Black, and Craig Kallendorf have offered detailed examinations of the depth of elementary education in Renaissance Italy.[29] While the quality of instruction in elementary schools varied according to the skills of the teachers, the many boys (and the few girls) who completed the roughly eight years of elementary education that commenced around the age of five would have acquired the ability to read and write in the vernacular, at least a passing familiarity with antiquity's more famous authors, and usually a basic knowledge of Latin.[30] As Paul Gehl has taught us, moreover, in Florence elementary education already exhibited these characteristics in the Trecento.[31] Craig Kallendorf has been especially attentive to one ubiquitous teaching tool in sixteenth-century Venice, the poetry of Virgil (especially the *Aeneid*), revealing its use in schools as a medium through which teachers might inculcate in their young students the values of traditional morality and a reverence for the political stability understood to derive from a rigid social hierarchy.[32] As these scholars all concede, however, general claims about reading in any given school or locality, let alone concerning what students working with tutors outside formal structures might have learned, can never encompass the diversity of evidence that particular cases yield. We also do well to consider the multiform literacies in premodern Europe that Armando Petrucci and others continue to elucidate.[33]

The account books of the Spinelli family, Venetian traders working in Cyprus, provide unusually detailed evidence of what students from a merchant family of the sixteenth century learned. Reading this ledger we get a better sense of what mercantile testators, especially if they had some discretionary income, meant when they spoke of educating their children. Agostino Spinelli often took charge of the sons of his brother Gasparo, and his account book running 1534–1549 details his expenses for the education of these four boys—expenses that included payments to teachers of *abbaco* (the practical mathematics that merchants would need for keeping accounts) and of the liberal arts, together with smaller sums for books, pens, paper, and ink.[34] The salaries of the teachers constituted the substantial investment of about eleven ducats per month, not counting other emoluments of wine and supplies for the school that students were expected to give their instructors. Especially interesting for our purposes, Spinelli allocated funds to his young relations earmarked for books. In 1549 alone, Spinelli set aside almost three ducats for the purchase, variously, of copies of Terence, Ovid, Erasmus, Pescennio Francesco Negro's treatise on Latin letter writing *(De modo epistolandi)*, a Donatus (the traditional Latin grammar book), and a compendium of moral philosophy, the *Fior di virtù*.

Spinelli's pedagogical expenses suggest that he may have intended to prepare the boys for different occupations: Gerolemo and Marchio studied primarily with a teacher of *abbaco*, but they also received some tutoring from a parish priest named Lauro; Zuanne and Bernardo studied the humanities at a grammar school. We might suspect that Gerolemo was being trained for an ecclesiastical career, as a parish priest played a considerable if not dominant role in his tuition and it was Gerolemo who bought the *Fior di virtù*. By contrast, Zuanne may have been aimed toward a civil profession that would have necessitated humanistic studies; he went to the grammar school, and the books that he bought were copies of Erasmus and Negro, which would have prepared him to writing Latin epistles. Marchio's purchase of a Donatus, however, reminds us that family strategies for children's future careers could be flexible: studying with an *abbaco* teacher might indicate that he was being encouraged to follow his father and uncle as a merchant, but his education in basic Latin grammar would also have provided a foundation for a career as a notary or almost any other profession. Spinelli does not tell us which of the boys purchased the Terence or the Ovid.

While we cannot be sure about the specific careers toward which these boys' readings were directed, we see another merchant family's serious commitment to humanistic learning. A secondhand goods dealer borrowing classical material becomes even less surprising in light of the literary studies prioritized in the Spinelli household, even if these young men do not seem to have undertaken Greek studies. While accounting constituted an important part of schooling for two of the children, the humanities were equally emphasized. Three of the boys learned Latin, and Zuanne must have attained an intermediate level of skill. Even if the Erasmus text that Zuanne purchased was the *Colloquies,* a lively and often comical book used in grammar schools (until the collected works of Erasmus appeared in the Index of Prohibited Books following the Council of Trent) to help young readers reach Latin proficiency, it would still have required Zuanne to be comfortable with the language.

The Spinelli family, then, much like the other Venetian men and women of middling rank, harbored both mercantile and cultural ambitions. Agostino was prepared to invest a great deal in literary skills no less than in commercial ones. These documents, then, like household inventories and wills, problematize the standard opposition scholars pose between literature and occupational reading.[35]

What prompted a merchant to fund the literary education of his younger relatives? Any merchant family, whether an ordinary one like Spinelli's or an extraordinary one like the Medici—or, for that matter, like most of Venice's governing elite, whose wealth lay more often in trade than land—had to confront the taint of lucre that remained a sociocultural liability. Spinelli did not have the resources to fund vast translation projects or build a neoclassical palazzo, routes to burnish their images that the wealthiest had at their disposal. But Spinelli and men of his station could prove their cultural legitimacy in more modest ways. At the most pragmatic level, giving children a humanistic education diversified the next generation's career prospects. As Brian Maxson and other scholars working on humanism and professional life have found, by the late fifteenth century a literary education served as an asset on a young man's curriculum vitae for a variety of government posts, even though, as Elizabeth McCahill demonstrates, navigating the humanist job market could sometimes involve as many obstacles as opportunities.[36] For those who were not seeking high positions civic government or the papal curia, however, a grammar-school education and university studies amply served to situate the recipient and their family among the cultural "right sort."

The same fusion of cultural and social aspirations informs the more laconic pedagogical instructions found, for instance, in the will of a glassblower named Martini Testa. Testa had no living children, but he had taken an interest in his nephew, Francesco, whom he had "raised as [his] own son." Testa put his cash where his rhetoric was, stipulating that all of his possessions should be sold, the proceeds invested, and the dividends used to "pay Francesco's teacher and then to support Francesco at the Academy of Salo until he earns his doctorate."[37] This glassblower aimed high; while his occupation had brought him a comfortable living, he hoped to situate his nephew and adoptive son in a different social rank. Bypassing two social levels would require, as Testa understood, not only a good grammar-school education but also a doctorate.

While less ambitious than Testa, a pharmacist's wife named Andriana articulated her own concern about and hopes for the education of a boy whom she and her husband had taken into their household and who probably also worked in their *bottega.* "For the love of God," Andriana urges, "I want Marco, whom we have at present in our house, to be kept there and I want him to be taught to read by my husband." She specified that her husband, Alessandro, should continue to protect and tutor this Marco "for four or five years."[38] Like Testa, Andriana and her husband seem not to have had any biological children but, also like Testa, she took a keen interest in equipping an adoptive heir with skills crucial for his future life and career. Andriana did not enjoin the young man to get a university degree, but she did want him to read well. Four or five years indicates the significant amount of time and energy she wanted her husband to expend on Marco's education. The verb *leggere* that Andriana used, moreover, tended not to indicate mere practical or occupational literacy but instead, as Ronald Witt has taught us, encompassed full command of reading and writing, at least in the vernacular.[39]

A Genoese merchant resident in Venice, Giacomo Cotre, invested even more intensely in the honor of a serious education: He made the education of his youngest son, Lorenzo, a formal condition of Lorenzo's patrimony.[40] Noting that Lorenzo was currently at his studies, Cotre sets aside an allowance of two hundred ducats to be paid quarterly over the next three years "to support his studies in one of the public academies in Italy." If Lorenzo should decide to terminate his academic endeavors, however, the penalty would be effective disinheritance. Cotre's system of values was not unique to himself or to his socioeconomic rank. A self-described Venetian "citizen" called Francesco Brognol also made education a condition of inheritance for his intended heir, the son of one of his cousins. Brognol informs this cousin, Hieronimo, that he is willing to bequeath his estate to Hieronimo's son on condition that Hieronimo name the boy "Zuanne Brognol" and make him study "the arts, that is, medicine."[41]

These exhortations about education and study put into sharp relief the social stakes of pedagogical endeavors for men and women outside the patriciate. We have seen artisans, merchants, priests, and physicians practicing testamentary humanism. As with book ownership, however, physicians once again stand out among these cultural aspirants. The testaments of medical doctors evince a striking insistence on cultural legitimacy. Indeed, physicians' pedagogical bequests would better be termed *humanistic hectoring.*

In a more agonistic vein than Father Pincio or Nicolò Paruta, the physician Valerio Superchio threatened his sons in his will of 1540, demanding that they succeed academically on pain of disinheritance. The connection between achievement and social mobility was clear to Superchio, who disinherited his eldest son, Gerolemo, for poor academic progress and general licentiousness. Gerolemo had entered the clerical life, receiving benefices at his father's expense. But since the boy had disappointed both in his studies and in his "vocation," Superchio rants, "I do not want him to have anything from my estate. And if he enters into some mad frenzy as bad priests usually do (obviously I am not talking about the good ones), paying no heed to the rule of poverty, his own youth, the costs of litigation, and the demands of legitimacy—in that case, even if the laws are against me, I will that he be compelled to repay the money that he has made me waste on his education. This money has only funded his libertine way of life (I refrain from saying anything worse to save his face) and amounts to more than 500 ducats in four years." Superchio's favored sons, Tiberio, Alessandro, and Ascanio, were to divide his estate equally, but only on condition, he explains, that they get along with each other and that they follow the career paths he has laid out for them: "Tiberio to a doctorate in medicine, Alessandro to a doctorate in law, and Ascanio to a doctorate in whatever subject he seems most inclined to pursue."[42] Valerio Superchio saw his sons as continuations of his own achievements, and the vehicles for the accumulation of more intellectual honor.

In his paternal rage against wasted academic opportunities, Superchio had much in common with the famous patrician humanist who would provide the epitaph for Superchio's headstone, Cardinal Pietro Bembo.[43] As adumbrated earlier, Bembo spent years threatening to disinherit his illegitimate son, Torquato, for poor academic performance.[44] As a patrician, Bembo had less to fear than Superchio in terms of making things work for his "natural" children. Still, Superchio and Bembo shared the problem of how to compensate for the obstacle that illegitimacy posed. For both men, intellectual cachet presented a solution, but this was all the more important for Superchio, whose children faced problems both of social status and of illegitimacy.

Even physicians who were not as anxious as Superchio hint that their bequests related to the continued social and cultural progress of their recipients. Maffeo dei Maffei, a prior of the College in 1529 and 1540, specified in his will of 1563 that if his grandsons wished to study, then his estate should be rearranged to fund their endeavors.[45] By implication, then, if these grandsons did not pursue degrees, the estate would not benefit them. Physicians' wives and medical practitioners of other sorts also participated in the spirit of insistent quests for cultural legitimacy. Maddalena Quattrocchi, widow of the physician Alberto Quattrocchi, freighted her bequest of a ruby ring worth twenty-five ducats to her son Bartolomeo with academic expectation. Signora Quattrocchi instructed her executors to give the ring to Bartolomeo only when he took his doctorate.[46] And a barber-surgeon called Philippo invested in his nephew's education, promising his brother an expensive bolt of cloth on condition that his brother's son would learn to read and write.[47] Once again, we see testators aiming to enhance their family's cultural legitimacy by citing its tradition, however recently inaugurated, of membership in the ranks of "uomini da bene."

TESTIFYING LITERARY AND ETHICAL COMMITMENTS

If testators making issues of books and education situated themselves and their families as people of the right sort, all the more so did those who seized the discursive opportunities latent in the "testament." In just over three thousand testaments, only two individuals cited a literary source. The career humanist Francesco Sansovino paused in his will of 1582 to forbid his executors to waste money in providing a lavish funeral for him. Elaborate funeral processions, Sansovino explains, "are neither necessary nor advisable, being nothing more than worldly pomp and vanity, as Saint Augustine attests."[48] Francesco Longo, a physician, in both his extant wills drew examples from Plutarch to teach his heirs about unanimity and magnanimity.[49] Lectures in Christian Stoicism as much as practical documents, Longo's remarkable testaments take center stage in Chapter 3. But there was more to testamentary humanism than direct literary references.

Natalie Zemon Davis and others have read early-modern Jewish wills as literature, especially as repositories of self-writing, a mode of analysis that we would do well to apply in other contexts.[50] A paradigmatic ethical will is that of Rabbi Leon of Modena, a Venetian by adoption, who appended his 1647 will to his autobiographical *Life of Judah.* Modena's testament adduces many of the same themes as his autobiography, making declarations about his priorities that emphasize his cultural and specifically literary merits. "I have no wealth or riches in my home to dispose of," Modena insists, "for it is empty and lacking in everything, praised be God. My everlasting gift is my written works: compositions, sermons, commentaries, and novellas of different kinds, all in great number."[51] Historians have traditionally read Christian wills for family history and social networks revealed by the transmission of property and legal responsibilities, but the work of Stanley Chojnacki, Caroline Castiglione, and Samuel Cohn have more recently taught us that wills are also archives of emotion, repositories of evidence about affection, disaffection, the constraints and opportunities of gender paradigms and lived religion.[52] These fruitful modes of reading, however, have not encompassed literary or philosophical questions. But Christian testators did sometimes echo what seems to have been a common practice for Jewish testators; they disposed of their souls and real property discursively, telling us portions of their life histories, signaling their intellectual priorities, and sometimes hinting at the ethical systems that animated and governed their lives.

While testaments cannot be seen as autobiography in the modern sense of coherent articulations of an autonomous individuality situated within a discrete literary genre, moments of idiosyncratic expressivity within them do constitute a historically significant form of writing. As many scholars have elucidated, our concept of autobiography would have been foreign to early-modern men and women, who worked within social, cultural, and literary constraints particular to their own time and place. Yet we have also learned in recent years to appreciate the diverse modes of "self-writing" that emerge in early-modern diaries, letters, and legal documents no less than in works entitled "lives" or biographies.[53] Thus, while early-modern records do not offer transparent expressions of subjectivities and experiences, they do contain representations of self that teach us a great deal about how historical actors worked within and around cultural norms and ideals.

Renaissance Venetians found many ways to craft images of themselves and the lives of their minds outside the formal mechanisms of publication; among their more creative choices were ethical bequests. Practitioners of testamentary humanism expatiated on unanimity, fortitude, industry, and accomplishment—*virtù* in the classical sense. In textual spaces designed for Christian exhortations, some testators also left philosophical gifts salutary for living well, and for ensuring an honorable posthumous reputation.

A common theme among ethically minded testators was that quintessential virtue of Venetian humanism: unanimity.[54] A priest, a lawyer, and two physicians organized their testaments around this ideal. Father Giovanni Soliero begged his three nephews (his principal heirs) to "live together in peace and goodwill," contenting themselves with the little that he is able to leave them.[55] Similarly, the lawyer Leo de Nigris asked his brother to accept in good grace the role of executor and residuary of his own small estate. In the course of this request, Nigris even traces the conceptual contours of brotherhood. "From the moment of my birth to this day," Nigris explains, "I have lived in a state of love and openness and fraternity with my brother, Lorenzo."[56] Nigris's formulation had both classical and Christian resonances. He acknowledges in "fraternity" the simple blood tie that, since antiquity, had been understood as a formal bond entailing reciprocal obligations. In mentioning "openness," Nigris invoked the conception of fraternity that had, from at least Aristotle onward, served as the defining hermeneutic of friendship: the principal duty of friends was to advise each other freely and openly, in the way of brothers.[57] Indeed, friendship and brotherhood had long served as metaphors for each other in philosophical discourse. By referring also to "love," Nigris weaves into this already complex framework the emotional dimension of friendship that linked both to the classical tradition and to Christian conceptions of *caritas*.

The physician Maffeo dei Maffei also emphasized love in addition to the more formal obligations of brotherhood, expressing his hope that his nephews "will be moved to love each other, as good brothers do," even if the younger should also pay to the elder "the respect due to older brothers."[58] Maffei's colleague, Nicolò Massa, had a more unwieldy collection of kin whom he hoped by testamentary exhortations to forge into a unity. There was his principal heir and executor, his illegitimate daughter, Maria. To assist and protect her, Massa enlisted his two nephews: Apollonio, a physician, and Lorenzo, a civil servant. Massa enjoins all three executors to "love one another and live together in peace and tenderness, helping each other as brothers and sisters do, with the peace of God and Jesus Christ."[59] Exhortations to unity usually accompany the standard anti-litigation clause whose purpose was practical. Yet reflections on the power and meaning of fraternity (or siblinghood) had a higher purpose. At the level of the city, the rhetoric of unity sought to transform an unstable collectivity into a cohesive polity. At the individual level, the same exhortations aimed to inspire the metamorphosis of accidental sanguinary ties into emotional and indeed sacred unions.

Our practitioners of testamentary humanism also reflect with remarkable eloquence on the values of self-determination and industry. These expressions of striving, including intellectual striving, belonged to a genealogy of ideas emergent in the fifteenth century, notably in the writings of Angelo Poliziano, which made the hallmark of the true philosopher competence in all disciplines—a reconceptualization that formed part of a larger revaluation of different types of work.[60] Heirs at least in a general way to this process of revaluation, two priests, one lawyer, and three physicians emphasized the virtue of dedication to many difficult things, even if they did not always have precisely Poliziano's interdisciplinarity in mind. Massa spoke of the value of effort in the first person, representing himself in his testaments no less than in his published works as a self-made man of letters, a problem we will explore in detail in Chapter 3. For the moment, it is important to note that the words to which Massa frequently returns in describing the process of building his life and nurturing his kin, supporting their educations and furthering their careers are "fatiche, affani et spesa" (toil, hassles and expense). As he moved toward the conclusion of his first attempt at a will, a forty-page draft written in 1562, Massa congratulated himself on his self-determination: "I am a debtor to no one. That which I leave my heirs is mine free and clear, earned by me and, as I've just said, I owe nothing to anyone—anyone at all—save, of course, my Lord God Eternal, from whose infinite generosity I realize derive all my possessions of mind and body alike, as well as my property and wealth. But these goods have also been accumulated thanks to my own extensive and zealous labor." Massa explains that the restitution of his mother's dowry took all that remained of his father's small estate, and so he was left (or so he claims) to make his way and to situate his family honorably using only his own talent and industry.[61]

This emphasis on industry and self-determination much earlier in the century and among different professional groups. A lawyer named Nicolò Paruta began his autograph will of 1544 citing his infelicitous family history as the spur to finish his testament in good time. "The fact that I suffered the ill-effects of paternal negligence," Paruta explains, "makes me cautious and serves as a continual spur lest, by delaying, I should fall into the same error. And so I, Nicolò Paruta, son of messer Andrea, have decided (with the help of God omnipotent, creator and prime mover of everything that exists) to make my testament and final will before death (which we pitiable mortals can never predict) strikes me unaware—and so that the little estate, which I have acquired with the help of God and my own industry and which I have conserved with great parsimony, may not be dissipated, but instead enjoyed (as I will arrange in due course) by those who live on after me as a memento of my labors and vigils."[62] Like Massa, Paruta insists that what little estate he has built derives from the combination of divine assistance and his own "exhausting efforts and vigils."

Venetian clerics also exalted the virtue of *virtù*. The parish priest of San Jacopo (Rialto), Federico Leon, began his autograph will of 1576 by noting that he had decided to make a testament of "that little estate granted to me by God together with my own hard work in teaching and celebrating humane letters."[63] His colleague, Paolo Pincio, also emphasized his years toiling in cultural fields. "At the age of fifty-seven," Pincio begins his own autograph will of 1597, "with a spirit as burdened with the many and harrowing worries that no human life can avoid as my body is worn out from the continual vigils and labors of my studies, I am reminded that it will not be long now before that day arrives when my most merciful lord God demands that I depart from this way-station we call mortal life and I must cease to be that which, thanks to Him, I have been until now."[64] Later in the will, Pincio bequeaths to his "sweetest and dearest Filippo," his illegitimate son, the entirety of his study, terming it "a memento of my vigils, so that you will come to know how I have acquired all that of which you now find yourself the heir—because I never had anything from my father or my mother other than my mere existence."[65]

The physicians Alvise Bognolo and Giovanni Battista Peranda took God out of the equation altogether, stating that they built their little worlds themselves, through their own effort. Bognolo, returning to Venice in August 1576 as the plague abated, notes his intention to put in order "what I wish to happen regarding the little by way of livelihood that I have gained through honorable labor."[66] Peranda is a bit more specific about that labor, observing his intention that "the estate which I now possess, acquired through my medical practice, and with much labor and sweat as well, be arranged after my death according to my wishes."[67]

This emphasis on honorable work, building an estate through intellectual and professional exertion, had a particular resonance for people in the midlands of the social landscape, people in motion and proud of their effortful activities and successes. This emphasis on exertion runs contrary to the prevalent concept of *sprezzatura* popularized by Baldassare Castiglione in *The Courtier*. Castiglione puts forward the ideal of the omnicompetent "Renaissance" individual: a person not only versed in the "noble" arts of warfare and politics but also skilled in (or at least conversant with) literature, music, and art. For all the work that would necessarily be involved in acquiring omnicompetence, however, the ideal courtier is never to suggest strain; they must retain an air of nonchalance *(sprezzatura)*, performing even the most difficult feats as if they were easy and feigning complete concentration on the tasks themselves, rather than on the reactions of their audiences.[68] Nonchalance may have been the favored posture at court, but the city had a different code. Our aspirants to cultural legitimacy of the urban middling ranks made the toil that funded their accomplishments a point of pride.

Testators who represented themselves as self-made also departed from common modes of narrating family history. A more usual approach would have been to invoke (or invent) the precedent set by some meritorious progenitor. Given the constant turmoil on the peninsula, there was nothing shameful in admitting that a family had fallen on hard times, and that one was working to "rebuild." Indeed, patriarchs and matriarchs of Renaissance Italy regularly urged their children to do just that. A fifteenth-century merchant widow named Alessandra Strozzi, much read in today's classrooms, insisted in her letters to her eldest son, Filippo, that it was his responsibility to reestablish his family in Florentine society in the wake of his father's exile and the Strozzis' subsequent political and financial hardships.[69]

This preoccupation with the value of industry also echoes the dichotomy between Fortuna and *virtù* ubiquitous in Renaissance discourse. One finds this polarity in humanist treatises, most famously Machiavelli's *The Prince*, but also in merchants' letters and accounts and in a bewildering array of visual images, as Aby Warburg, Ernst Cassirer, and Erwin Panofsky showed long ago.[70] Still, confronting adversity to preserve or reestablish an honorable lineage was one thing; constructing it from the ground up was another.

A few patricians also devoted space in their wills to encouraging virtuous endeavor, but they wrote of these matters in different terms. Patricians did not use the word *sweat*, as Peranda did, nor did they speak of their estates as products of hassles and headaches as Massa and others did. Patricians had hassles and headaches, too, but in their milieu mentioning effort was indecorous. Consider the nobleman Lorenzo Donaldo, who devoted the last paragraphs of his ten-folio will to counseling his then five-year-old son, Alvise, and bequeathing to him a gift of a father's worldly wisdom. "Believe me, I know what I am talking about," Donaldo insists, "thanks to the experience I have amassed over the course of many years and my encounters with (I suppose I can say) all the ways of the world." Donaldo urges Alvise to attend to his studies and to acquire knowledge of "good letters" (that is, the humanities), but he does not construe their acquisition as the means by which estate and honor may be built. Rather, he situates literary studies as the servant of piety and, in particular, a necessary diversion from the vice of gambling. His son should study, first and foremost, so that he might comprehend better "the holiest mysteries of the Mass," reasoning that "to hear the Mass but not understand it is of little use to our souls." Later in the will, Donaldo once again enjoins Alvise to study literature (this time adding the study of music), but he terms these occupations "honorable pastimes and pleasures" *(tratenimenti et piaceri honoreveli),* diversions that would, he hoped, leave his son no time for the ruinous vice of gambling. The danger Donaldo hoped to avert through his instructions was decadence, not lack of wherewithal or a bulwark against the inroads of potential enemies. Alvise need not sweat to make his fortune or build a reputation; he need only divert himself to avoid dissipating the financial and cultural capital he would naturally inherit.[71]

At best, patrician testators represented education as the means by which their heirs would acquire social graces. Marc'Antonio Zantani, for instance, urges his executors to support his son Hieronymo "at the school of the liberal arts until he becomes reasonably proficient in letters (something they should do for any other son that I might produce) . . . and similarly the girls should be brought up to have the finest manners."[72] In Zantani's view, academic preparation (for the boys) and manners (for the girls) conferred polish. Zantani did not give either enterprise the urgency or significance that testators in less exalted social ranks did. Certainly, Hieronymo was not to be pushed his education, as he need only acquire a "sufficiency" of literary grace. Another patrician, Antonio Diedo, similarly wedged literary studies between manners and morality. Diedo instructs his executors to make his sons learn "good manners, letters, and, above all, the fear of God" until the boys turned nineteen, further specifying that he wished his sons to be kept "in the Academies outside the city of Venice."[73] For Diedo, education meant containment, "keeping" his sons in the Academies and away from Venice; by contrast, our glassblower Martini Testa insisted that his entire estate should be sold to "support" his adoptive heir's doctoral studies. This is not to suggest that Donaldo or Diedo misapplied education when they attempted to use it to shield their heirs from the city's potentially dissipating entertainments. Yet it is striking that the lower we go on the social scale, the more intellectual attainments mentioned in wills come closer to echoing humanists' idealistic rhetoric, and, conversely, the higher on the social scale we go the more testators give the same attainments mere ornamental or prophylactic value.

ASSESSING VENICE'S TESTAMENTARY HUMANISTS

Stepping back, what general picture can we form of Venice in the late Renaissance drawing on these book bequests, provisions for education, and ethical excurses exhorting unanimity, industry, and *virtù*? Were humanistic testators representative of the cultural ferment extending through their society, or were they actually outliers? To be sure, passionate concern for cultural matters cannot be considered normative any more than we could claim that secondhand goods dealers usually borrowed manuscripts of Greek philosophy. That said, the social and occupational ordinariness of messer Francesco and of the majority of our testamentary humanists militates against classifying these individuals as exceptional. Let us put a number to the problem. On the one hand, out of my 3,005 wills only forty-six testators (less than 2 percent of the group) articulate one or more of the themes of testamentary humanism. On the other hand, testators who took a humanistic turn worked against the grain, departing from the definition of the will as a disposition of one's soul and property. Indeed, the would-be testamentary humanist had to overcome explicit legal injunctions forbidding idiosyncratic expression in this medium.

The Udinese lawyer, jurist, and cardinal Francesco Mantica (1534–1614) wrote the most influential compendium of knowledge on making a will, *De coniecturis ultimarum voluntatum*. In this monumental tome, Mantica offered his notarial readers copious advice, including how to avoid "the vice of superfluity."[74] Notaries must ensure clarity by refraining from excess verbiage of their own and keeping their clients on task, that is, bequeathing their souls to God, bequeathing their most valuable property to their principal heirs, specifying their executors, and making their charitable bequests. One suspects, then, that some testators who might otherwise have been inclined to say more or different things yielded to the discursive curfew of their notaries, if not to the two even stronger countervailing pressures, illness and time.

Given these circumscriptions, it makes sense that a third of our humanistic testators (fourteen individuals) wrote wills in their own hands, thereby enabling themselves to "testify" according to their own priorities and in their own words. It is surprising, however, that a range of testators across the urban social categories wrote autograph wills, not just the university-trained men whom we might have assumed would be most likely to take pen in hand. More interesting still, the impulse to talk about books, education, or "virtue" in the non-Christian sense correlated almost inversely to status. Patricians were no more likely to make book bequests or to philosophize than parish priests were.[75] In fact, patricians were far less likely to take a humanistic turn than physicians. Self-described "citizens," men of sub-patrician rank whose disavowal of a particular occupation at least rhetorically distanced them from the mercantile world, constitute only two cases. By contrast, five unabashed retail merchants went the humanistic route. And artisans even edged beyond humanistic testators of citizen rank by a tiny margin.

As with book ownership, cases of testamentary humanism confirm some reasonable expectations. Testators with university degrees loom large among those who chose to emphasize their intellectual honor. Indeed, university-educated men constitute 43 percent of humanistic testators. We might also assume that artisans and retail merchants would be less likely than priests, lawyers, or physicians to make book bequests or to talk about education, and this is the case. Yet it tells us something about the breadth of the quest for cultural legitimacy that artisans and merchants appear at all, let alone constitute (together) 17 percent of the group.

A further surprise emerges when we consider humanistic wills in terms of their frequency by professional category. The most celebrated humanists—Leonardo Bruni, Thomas More, Pietro Bembo, Michel de Montaigne—were most often affiliated with government, law, or the church. Accordingly, we might have expected either lawyers or priests to claim pride of place among practitioners of testamentary humanism. Instead, physicians and their kin dominate. Fourteen people associated with the medical profession (twelve physicians and two physicians' wives) took literary turns in their wills, thus representing one-third of our humanistic testators. Eight priests and eight patricians also wrote distinctly literary-minded testaments—a good showing but far less impressive than our physicians. The remainder of these humanistic testators represent a scattering of the urban occupations: six lawyers, five merchants, two "citizens," and three artisans. This prevalence of physicians is all the more impressive when we take into account that these men and their kin, demographically speaking, constituted a tiny minority. Physicians, it seems, were particularly eager to leave some trace of their intellectual ambitions and accomplishments.

Physicians also asserted their literary priorities in greater depth and complexity than most other groups. Redistributing our forty-six humanistic testators across the three criteria of discussion of books, remarks about education, and reflections on ethics and *virtù,* we find that only four testators emphasized all three themes. Two of these emphatically humanistic testators were the physicians Nicolò Massa and Giovanni Battista Peranda; the other two were the parish priests Federico Leon and Paulo Pincio.[76] Physicians also constitute eight of the fifteen testators who made two of these three humanist planks components of their wills. The others in this category include two priests, two lawyers, one patrician, one merchant, and one artisan.[77] Physicians (together with parish priests) also distinguished themselves among the twenty testators who made book bequests. Eight medical doctors and seven priests talk about books in the course of their wills.[78] It is rare to find any other category of testator considering a library in this context. Only two patricians, two lawyers, and one merchant mentioned texts; no "citizens" or artisans did so.[79] The topic of education involved the most diverse roster of people, but physicians once again set themselves apart. Physicians' regular attention to pedagogical ideals and the transmission of their intellectual honor again suggests pressing commitments. Eleven physicians discussed education in their wills.[80] Artisans, retail merchants, "citizens," lawyers, priests, and patricians were less consistent, but two to three individuals in each of these groups still voiced a commitment to education.[81]

A representative sampling of testators also discussed ethics or *virtù*. As in the case of book bequests, however, physicians narrowly surpassed priests in the frequency with which they made ethical or philosophical bequests. Six physicians maximized the discursive potential of the testament; five priests did the same.[82] But artisans, merchants, lawyers, and patricians also occasionally paused in the midst of their dispositions of property to consider virtues such as industry and unanimity, or their families' intellectual and professional honor. Between one and three individuals in each of these groups took this form of the humanistic turn.[83]

The practitioners of testamentary humanism, then, although a smaller group than Venetian book owners, nonetheless mirror their social distribution. While patricians discussed books or ethics rarely, artisans, merchants, professionals, and above all physicians did so more regularly. Much as Matthew Lundin argues concerning his writerly Cologne lawyer, there indeed seems to be a connection between reading, writing, and what Lundin terms the "anxieties of upward mobility."[84] Hermann Weinsberg both benefited and suffered from his family's movement from the artisanal and mercantile ranks to positions of some civic prominence. Weinsberg's father, Christian, worked as a wine merchant, but reading Cicero's *De oratore,* together with Livy, Herodotus, Plutarch, and Justinian in his thirties inspired new sociocultural ambitions. Weinsberg the elder leveraged positions for himself in local government and shoved the (unfortunately mediocre) talents of young Hermann toward academic endeavor in the same way we have seen Venetian testamentary humanists doing.[85]

Animated by their quest for cultural legitimacy, men and women in the middle ranks of Venetian society collected books and sometimes creatively appropriated the expressive potential of that melancholy and altogether unpleasant document, the final will and testament. Put another way, Venetians left traces of books and learning everywhere. But the traces gleaned through inventories and wills suggests a desire characteristic of the urban artisanal, mercantile, and professional worlds to prove engagement with intellectual and literary concerns. This form of concern with reputation motivated the people who were close to yet still outside the ranks of those assumed to possess the highest merit. While the lending records of the Marciana reveal only one mercantile borrower, the legal records of the Archivio di Stato bring us many figures eager to prove their worth in terms other than finance.

Of all the occupational groups we have encountered, however, physicians emerged as the most consistent practitioners of testamentary humanism. The urge to bequeath books, educate relatives, and leave ethical bequests we see in the cases of medical doctors and their kin parallel what we have already learned about their voracious book collecting. These commitments, together with physicians' frequent demands for further intellectual social mobility from their heirs, suggest a peculiar eagerness (even overeagerness) to claim cultural legitimacy. It is time, then, to examine more closely the lives, careers, fears, and aspirations of physicians as they confronted and sometimes broke through the marble ceiling of Renaissance Venice's sociocultural elite.

PART II

CHAPTER 3

NICOLÒ MASSA, A SELF-MADE MAN OF LETTERS

Nicolò Massa was among the few physicians to draw notice in Francesco Sansovino's popular two-volume synopticon of Venetian excellence, *Delle cose notabili della città di Venetia.* In a section devoted to Venice's leading philosophers and theologians, Sansovino praises Massa as "a celebrated physician and philosopher of exceedingly broad wisdom." Massa contributed to the common good through publishing accessible works on preventative medicine, Sansovino notes, but immediately thereafter he assures his readers that this medical doctor also "wrote other works of philosophy and logic, which I know you will have seen as they are so widely in circulation that nearly everyone has a copy."[1] This tribute is singular: Massa is the only medical doctor on whom Sansovino lavishes so much as a sentence. The other physicians to whom he refers appear in a perfunctory list of urban professionals.[2] What might have led Sansovino to favor Nicolò Massa, a recognized member of Venice's College of Physicians but a minor figure in the medical community compared with his contemporary Vettore Trincavella? Part of the answer lies in Massa's prolific authorship. Sansovino exaggerated in claiming that "nearly everyone" had copies of Massa's publications, which constituted specialist works in Latin and within the genre of medical humanism. Nonetheless, Massa's works brought him a considerable professional and student audience. And, more fundamental for enhancing his wider reputation, Massa expended tremendous energy courting the approbation of literary arbiters such as Sansovino.

Massa repays attention not for his stature but for his struggles. Having earned certification first as a surgeon, Massa specialized in anatomy and made a few refinements to Galenic medicine that Vesalius's techniques and discoveries instantly eclipsed. Accordingly, historians have traditionally made Massa a footnote to Vesalius. Richard Palmer began to change that, capitalizing on the rich collection of Massa family papers to elucidate the energy and skill with which this physician overcame poverty and a series of tragedies to build a household and ultimately a considerable estate.[3] Palmer also sketched Massa's distinctive persona as a "self-made" man, evident in his unpublished family papers no less than his print publications.[4] Palmer's purpose, ably fulfilled, was to demonstrate Massa's rags to riches story and to understand the connections between the catalysts of that story: Massa's medical practice and medical publications on the one hand, his real estate investments on the other. Following Palmer, Nancy Siraisi has recently unearthed Massa once again, using him not as an example of a physician accumulating financial capital in difficult circumstances but instead as one accumulating professional capital through strategic epistolary networking.[5]

Palmer's Massa exemplified the self-made man in economic terms. Siraisi's Massa emerges as the self-made professional man. I would like to complicate the picture, emphasizing that Massa's conception of his meritorious autonomy had as much to do with engaging the literary as it did with money, property, and professional clout. The Massa we find here is the self-made man of letters. "I am a debtor to no one," we have seen the old physician insist in his lengthy draft will of 1562. "That which I leave my heirs is mine free and clear, earned by me and, as I've just said, I owe nothing to anyone—anyone at all—save, of course, my Lord God Eternal, from whose infinite generosity I realize derive all my possessions of mind and body alike, as well as my property and wealth. But these goods have also been accumulated thanks to my own extensive and zealous labor."[6] As Palmer has shown, that "extensive and zealous labor" involved medical practice and publication, as well as shrewd investments. As Siraisi demonstrates, that labor also included effective letter campaigns. But Massa's conception of the mind as an asset went beyond financial and professional successes, meshing with the cultural dimension inherent in the idea of the *uomo da bene* other testamentary humanists articulated.

Through analysis of Massa's writings in print and manuscript as well as the people and texts prominent in his immediate milieu, the Venetian College of Physicians and contemporary reception of medicine as a field, we see Massa as representative of a particular moment in medicine's fraught relationship to literary culture. More broadly, this physician's fight to gain credibility for himself, his family, and his profession constitutes a representative case of the battle for honor in a late Renaissance urban world. Massa believed that neither money nor occupational success could bring him the cultural legitimacy that literary credentials did. To judge by Sansovino's approbation, Massa took the right approach.

THE CASE FOR MEDICINE AS A LIBERAL ART

From the beginning to end of his career, Nicolò Massa positioned his writing in medicine as philosophy and literature. We see his discursive labor in this regard with particular clarity in his consistently elaborate dedications, which situate the author, his profession, and the genre of medicine itself within the cultural field of the liberal arts. Massa makes even technical and practical texts not merely *ars* but *scientia*—and even *bonae litterae.* As an individual who began his career with no social distinction or connections, in dire financial distress, and holding only a barber-surgeon's certification, the projects of proving his own merit and that of practical medicine became mutually sustaining if not coterminous endeavors.

Even in his first publications, Nicolò Massa marshaled the art of the humanistic prefatory epistle to stake claims to cultural legitimacy for author and profession alike. Dedicating his *Liber introductorius anatomiae* (1536) to Pope Paul III, a canny choice as the patron of a manual on how to dissect human beings that had potentially objectionable spiritual ramifications, he construes the offering as a literary gift to the pontiff. While he writes in accessible Latin and references his own expertise in the operating theater, he positions the *Introduction* as his calling card to literary society. Just as diligent agriculturalists must tend a variety of fields to yield the best and most abundant produce, he argues, so intellectuals should cultivate a variety of literature to produce the most perfect compositions. Situating himself as just such an intellectual, he explains, "When I had already been zealously laboring in the medical field for a long time, I began to till literary fields and I preserved the sweet fruits I found there."[7]

Massa goes on to cite his practical experience in conducting dissections as a qualification for writing the book, but he manages to make these endeavors connect to the world of letters. Even his time in the anatomical theater, he insists, involved collaboration with men of letters, "other cultivators of the liberal arts, amongst whom His Magnificence Gerolemo Marcello, a most learned philosopher whom I have always considered my 'faithful Achates' and to whom I promised that I would write this little introductory text."[8] And although Massa also positions anatomical dissection as an improvement on the ancients, a way to know more (or different) things than they knew and in that sense practically useful to his contemporaries, he nonetheless ultimately positions his book as a literary contribution. "So take up these my labors, Most Blessed Father," he urges in concluding his dedication, "and look favorably upon them, so that I may be confirmed, under your protection, as a member of literary society and so that you may find me offering you even better and more abundant produce in the future."[9]

However smooth the elision between literary and medical endeavors in Massa's dedication, tensions persisted between the arts and sciences. If the late medieval rhetorical battles between physicians and rhetoricians seemed to have calmed, there had been no cease-fire let alone a conclusive peace. Massa's two-volume *Epistolarum medicinalium* (1558) dispenses eight hundred pages of diagnostic advice and analysis of the most common maladies through the medium of elegant Latin letters directed to patients, colleagues, and patrons. As Siraisi has urged, the letter collection as a genre deserves much more attention from historians of medicine than it has traditionally received, because letters embed at least three types of information. Certainly physicians' epistles present their medical knowledge; many of their letters were *consilia,* case studies or short treatises, masquerading as correspondence. Letters also reveal professional networks and even contain a measure of their authors' social history.[10] We do well to bear in mind, moreover, that medium itself sent a message. While the treatise hinted of scholasticism, the epistle marked the author as versed in the humanist way of packaging knowledge. Massa's decision to invest in the epistolary mode at the culmination of his career underscores his desire for humanistic credibility. But far from appearing in his letters a comfortable physician-humanist of the sort that Siraisi has found, he devotes considerable energy to polemics against rhetoricians and ardent defenses of his profession against literary detractors—calumniators, as he calls them.

The battle between physicians and rhetoricians emerges throughout Massa's encyclopedic collection of letters. But the stakes appear with particular clarity in his letter (dated 1556), "To All Scholars of the Good Arts and All True Lovers of Wisdom," an apologia for medicine's recognition as a humanistic discipline. Massa takes aim at the calumnies physicians suffer from contemporaries who claim to be grammarians or literary men—calumnies centered on the relative lack of eloquence in medical texts. Physicians are maligned, he complains, for doing what they should be doing, that is, writing clearly and comprehensibly in the service of human life not literary eloquence. But Massa also turns calumniators' criticisms against themselves, accusing literary authors of weakening their own prose with superfluities and rhetorical ornament. When discussing the most important and elevated subjects, he lectures, whether medicine or theology or poetry "there is no need to look for greater eloquence, because the greatest and most sublime things [. . .] are quite ornate and sophisticated enough in and of themselves. If elegance and style of writing consist in the most persuasive reasoning and use of the strongest evidence, as the wise always affirm, painting on rhetorical 'rouge' trivializes your subject instead of enhancing it. The same thing often happens to pretty women when they exert themselves in applying cosmetics to their faces; instead of enhancing their beauty, they spoil it."[11] Undermining the cultural authority of rhetoricians through accusations of irrelevance and even a suggestion of effeminacy, Massa likens medicine to theology and poetry, fields so inherently significant that they require discussion in a leaner style. Using excessive rhetoric in these fields, he suggests, prostitutes their serious content.

We might consider Massa's approach hypocritical, insofar as there is plenty of rhetoric in his own writing, including the analogy he has just used. But hypocrisy would not be quite the right characterization. Massa's argument echoes an internal contradiction characteristic of the literary world he hoped to join. His simultaneous disavowal and use of rhetoric had been a common tactic in literary writing since antiquity. And some of the most celebrated authors of the earlier Renaissance reflected at great (and eloquent) length on the issue. Consider, for instance, the *Lamia* of Angelo Poliziano (1454–1494), a tricky text recently disentangled for us by Christopher Celenza.[12] A rejoinder to university philosophers who had criticized Poliziano for overstepping his competencies as a grammarian by lecturing on their areas of expertise, especially Aristotle, Poliziano's barbed exposition highlights an opposition between content and form—in this case, between philosophy and literary eloquence—that had sparked debate for centuries.[13] At the same time, Poliziano offered a possible reconciliation by insisting that he, a rhetorician by training, had nonetheless read philosophy with sufficient rigor to teach the subject to undergraduates at least. In the end, Celenza argues, Poliziano expanded "the traditional province of the *grammaticus* to include all disciplines and in the end to be representative of the only true way of seeking wisdom."[14] We cannot be certain if Nicolò Massa read Poliziano's *Lamia,* but he shared Poliziano's animus against disciplinary boundaries and territorialism. Unlike Poliziano, however, as a physician Massa could claim full expertise neither as rhetorician nor as philosopher; thus he remained doubly excluded.

Given the cachet attached to eloquence in contemporary culture at large, Massa also had a particular need to fight rhetoricians using their own weapons. In so doing, he proved that he was not, as a medical doctor, incapable of elegance. Instead, Massa refused to mar the dignity of his subject with extraneous verbiage. In the terms he uses later in the essay, he resisted the "siren-song" of literary ornament in the service of fact, truth, and his readers' comprehension.[15] In short, Massa's polemical strategy was by no means original to himself, hearkening back as far as Plato (an authority he cites often) and the ancient battle of philosophy against poetry, and continuing into contemporary debates between university philosophers and rhetoricians. In Massa's professional context, however, new exigencies inflected these long-standing dichotomies of clarity and truth versus illusion and artifice.

The tensions in Massa's writing reveal that aspiring and even accomplished physician-intellectuals confronted a dilemma. They hoped to dignify themselves and their profession by proving their capabilities not just as competent philosophers and doctors of medicine but also as learned and eloquent writers worthy of membership in the humanist *res publica litterarum.* Yet literary superfluity displayed by men who were supposed to be focused on healing human bodies risked ridicule. Indeed, in the popular literature of the day physicians appear either as grasping, duplicitous mercenaries or as supercilious windbags. Master Mercurio in Pietro Aretino's *Il Cortegiano,* for instance, modeled the first type.[16] In Niccolò Machiavelli's *Mandragola,* the character Callimaco, disguised as a physician and using concatenations of Latin quips to dupe the childless, irascible, and gullible lawyer Nicia, merged elements of both stereotypes.[17]

In the world of print, there were three useful options for physicians to prove their literary worth without seeming to cultivate an ornamentation unsuited to their occupational objectives: translation and emendation projects; publishing literary works outside the field of medicine; and, blending the two, targeted literary excurses in medical texts. Vettore Trincavella, for example, took the first option; his complete works contain both his revisions of the Galenic corpus and an earlier translation from the Acts of the Apostles. Lorenzo Marucini favored poetry and local biography. Nicolò Massa took the third option, using his dedicatory letters and other prefatory material, together with select portions of his collected works, to do literary business and prove his refined sensibilities. When the topic was diagnosis and remedy, however, he stuck to the facts.

As a rule, Massa proved his humanistic learning in the process of praising his dedicatees for theirs. Indeed, Massa maximized the self-aggrandizing potential of the dedication, writing an individual epistle not only for each volume but also for each chapter within each volume. In dedicating his 1555 treatise on the plague to Elizabeth, Landgravin of Hesse, for instance, he informs her that in writing to her he has in mind the example of ancient authors, "who generally brought their writings into public view under the patronage of some (as they called him) Maecenas and from whom they derived both protection and greater authority."[18] Massa follows this classical compliment with another bit of literary flattery for Elizabeth's brother, Phillip, whom he characterizes as "almost another Achilles."[19]

The range of Massa's references underscore his literary self-fashioning. Massa was nearly as likely to cite Virgil, Homer, and Plato as he was Hippocrates or Galen. Massa also followed the time-honored practice of including in his prefatory material laudatory poems written by established authors, letting them do some of the literary talking for him.[20] His occasional dedication to a recognized literary celebrity also afforded the opportunity to make a claim to participation in their world. Massa's final essay in the *Epistolarum,* "On the Generation of Man and His Nobility," takes the form of a letter to the literary patron Bernardino Feliciano. From Pico della Mirandola's famous oration onward, the topic remained de rigueur for literary humanists. Massa's dedicatee was the son of the humanist pedagogue and patristic commentator Giovanni Bernardo Feliciano from whom (as Massa reminds Bernardino) Massa himself had once learned Greek.[21]

Massa thus found many ways of emphasizing his accomplishments in languages, literary forms, and even literary topics. As we have learned from Nancy Siraisi, many physicians wrote on topics other than medicine, especially history.[22] Kate Lowe has also contended that the methodological homology between the examination of medical and historical "cases" invited and shaped the distinctive contributions of physicians, as well as their learned daughters, to this humanistic discipline.[23] I am suggesting that we attend with equal care to physicians' less sustained but no less revealing moments of humanistic self-presentation within their medical writings as such. Physicians larded their works with literary references tangential to the subject, even considering the high standard for superfluous exempla in contemporary writing of all genres. The fraught quality of these humanistic habits suggests that medical doctors, despite their advanced educations, still campaigned for a position in literary culture.

Physicians waged their cultural campaign against multiple axes of suspicion. We have already considered the unfortunate figure of the physician in contemporary drama. But negative stereotypes also abounded in the academic genres physicians like Massa encountered on a regular basis. Even in the late sixteenth century, it still took considerable effort for a medical doctor to prove himself truly learned and thus honorable on the standards of literary humanism. Physicians of the late Renaissance still needed to address the charges that humanists had been leveling at them for centuries. One such accusation (or insult) was that physicians were manual laborers with delusions of grandeur. Petrarch had set the censorious paradigm in the fourteenth century, castigating medical doctors as mechanics and parvenus. "How can I believe that you are a philosopher," Petrarch asked one imagined physician-antagonist, "when I know you are a mercenary mechanic? I gladly repeat this term, since I know that no other reproach stings you more."[24] Good to his word, he inflicted ten more stings of the same type in this invective alone. Not only did Petrarch castigate physicians with a view toward exalting his own preferred "pure" life of the mind; he also cast in the worst possible light the opportunities for social advancement that the medical profession afforded.

To ennoble his art and bring himself honor, the physician had options in the realm of action and in the realm of rhetoric. A medical doctor could eschew remuneration, or try to rely on stipends from his college and possibly teaching fees, directing his medical services instead to the poor, working free of charge or for minimal honoraria.[25] But he would still, in the eyes of humanists, be essentially an artisan. He could also abandon, or reduce, his work as a medical practitioner, devoting himself instead to theoretical medicine. That is, he could put his university training to use in emending the classical medical corpus, or writing treatises and collections of *consilia* (advice) that might be publicly beneficial, as Vettore Trincavella and Nicolò Massa, among many others, did. If physicians engaged in literary work, as even acerbic Petrarch had conceded, they might be considered philosophers of a kind.

Physicians devised cunning and sometimes effective defense mechanisms, but their efforts remind us that Petrarchan criticism endured, even if in weakened form. On the one hand, Nancy Siraisi and George McClure have demonstrated that humanist praise of the medical profession and of individual physicians can be found in the fifteenth century and, even more so, in the sixteenth century. On the other hand, humanists who looked favorably on the medical profession weighted "the physician's task" (to borrow Siraisi's phrase) more toward intellectual or philosophical than toward practical labor.[26] Physicians, far more than lawyers, their nearest relatives on the professional family tree, found themselves uncomfortably positioned between artisanal work and a "civil profession." This problem was often exacerbated by physicians' social origins among the ranks of higher artisans, especially pharmacists.[27] In his popular encyclopedia of the world's occupations, Tommaso Garzoni archly situated physicians between butchers and theologians.[28]

Anxieties about social mobility through medical education and the taint of medicine's "mechanical" dimension that fueled Petrarch's animus in the fourteenth century lingered in the sixteenth century. In addition to Garzoni's *Piazza*, we have Fabio Glissenti's *Discorsi morali contra il dispiacere di morire, detto Athanatophilia* (Moralistic Dialogues against the Disinclination to Die, Otherwise Called the Love of Immortality, 1596). George McClure has analyzed Glissenti's dialogue with great sensitivity, but let us consider for a moment a passage that McClure does not discuss. Considering the city of Venice, one of Glissenti's principal interlocutors, a courtier, remarks to the other, a philosopher: "Every household [in Venice] has its 'professor,' everyone prides themselves on being knowledgeable, and there's no profession in this city more populous than that of medicine, which purports to extend life and health. Not only do university physicians, surgeons, barber-surgeons, midwives and charlatans want to take up this line of work, but so too every other vagrant. We can even include woodworkers, gondoliers, servants and similar folk, for whom it would be better to have an oar in hand than a doctor's razor which, if it is not applied skillfully, with knowledge, experience and discretion, at the right time, in the right place and with a degree of force calibrated to the patient's needs, wounds instead of healing, and instead of giving life causes Death."[29] Aware of the long-standing criticism of medical work as an avenue for laborers and artisans to climb the social ladder, Glissenti aimed to defend the profession. The courtier makes some concessions to medicine's critics by blaming incompetent practitioners. Yet he also praises the skill and knowledge possessed by those really proficient in the medical arts, the true physicians who are notable—mortally so—in their absence.

Glissenti had personal experience of the social and economic conflicts attendant to the field of health care. Although he only refers to his occupation allusively in his preface and he has no physician-speakers in the dialogue itself, Glissenti was himself a physician. Indeed, he would become prior of the College in 1601, a few years after the publication of his *Discorsi morali*.[30] More particularly, he was a physician who ennobled his profession by publishing morally edifying literature. His corpus of writings includes not only this monumental (six-hundred-folio) dialogue but also numerous editions of *favole morali* (moral tales) that brought the ongoing revival of classical moral philosophy to vernacular audiences. In this, his model may well have been the fifteenth-century Florentine humanist Leonardo Bruni, who spent much of his own career engaged in translating classical moral philosophy for Italian readers, as James Hankins has shown.[31] Aligning with such a recognizably humanistic project, Glissenti brought honor to his profession. As it turned out, the learned societies governing that profession used many of Glissenti's themes and rhetorical strategies. If Massa crafted the image of the man of letters, his college and its membership strove to prove not their required technical competence but their meritorious literary knowledge.

THE CULTURAL LEGITIMACY OF VENICE'S COLLEGE OF PHYSICIANS

The Venetian College of Physicians has long occupied the footnotes of histories tracing the so-called professionalization of medicine.[32] Like other institutions of its type, the Venetian College worked to establish a coherent occupational organization, to oversee the credentialing of new doctors, to regulate the activities of other medical workers (especially pharmacists and barber-surgeons), and to define and disseminate the best practices for healing. Richard Palmer has given the Venetian College a more prominent place on the scholarly map, arguing that it was not a "paper university" lurking in Padua's shadow but instead a rival institution.[33] Palmer highlights the College's vitality as a sodality for physicians with varied interests who published voluminous emendations of Aristotle and Galen and new treatises concerning surgery, botany, and pharmacology.[34]

Departing from Palmer's emphasis on the College's institutional history and its contributions to medical humanism as such, we will consider here this sodality's wider cultural priorities. Following Nancy Siraisi, Sandra Cavallo, and David Gentilcore, I take physicians' "occupational diversity," especially their commitment to the ideals of the liberal arts, not as extracurricular but instead as central to physicians' professional identities.[35] As Siraisi observes, Renaissance physicians' "bookish erudition encompassing not only medicine but also other humanistic fields was a major ingredient both in professional self-image and in professional success, as measured by such indicators as court patronage and evidences of wealth."[36] What was true for European physicians in general was certainly true for sixteenth-century Venetians in particular. Both the Venetian College as an entity and its individual members emphasized their humanistic ideals. We understand this institution best, then, by appreciating its cultural as much as its medical objectives. Even if this College did not rank with contemporary academies as a knowledge community, the physicians who congregated in it engaged in projects of literary self-presentation that ran parallel to and reinforced their medical endeavors and publications. These projects emerge in many collegiate' publications, but with special clarity in the defenses and celebrations of its members.

Physicians argued and competed in the usual way of academics, but they turned fraternal when one of their number came into difficulty, especially if the afflicted one had enhanced the College's prestige. Such was the case for Nicolò Massa. During his eighties, Massa suffered blindness in addition to a series of other calamities that would culminate in the death of a cherished grandson, who had just launched a promising legal career. As some measure of compensation for the particularly cruel blow of blindness, his colleagues, protégés, and admirers rallied to celebrate his indomitable virtue and the humanistic qualities of his life and work on which he himself insisted from his first publications to his last will and testament (of which more below).

Massa and the profession had in collegiate Alvise Luisin (Luigi Luisini) an especially clever and influential encomiast. Luisin's 1569 *Dialogue Entitled Blindness* (*Dialogo intitolato la cecità*), as Richard Palmer has pointed out, complimented and consoled the old doctor as he confronted affliction. Massa is the subject of the dialogue, and the conceit is that all the speakers, having just learned that their old friend has gone blind, decide to pay him a visit and bring him what cheer they can. The characters are modeled on Massa's kin and friends, from his ill-fated grandson Francesco Grifalconi (a secretary who died less than a year after this publication went to press) and his nephews (the physician Apollonio and Nicolò Crasso, a lawyer) to his closest medical colleagues, Alvise Luisin and Giovanni Martini.[37] Palmer reads this dialogue compellingly as evidence of Massa's reputation and career success. But I would add that we understand this text within the context of the humanistic cultural campaign common to the medical profession in late Renaissance Venice.

Luisin makes each character's speech a patchwork of literary references, but reserves the most exceptional performance for one of the physician speakers, "Apollonio Massa." In describing his uncle's blindness, "Apollonio" reaches not for diagnoses from Hippocrates or Galen, but instead provides citations of lost or weakened vision from the ancient literary canon. Perhaps exaggerated in the interest of amusing his readers, Luisin's decision to string together so many citations from ancient literature shows us again the literary special pleading at the heart of the campaign for respect waged by many physicians, including Massa. "Apollonio," when asked how his uncle came to his misfortune, launches into a disquisition on mythological and historical figures who went blind, from the seer Tiresias and singer Thamyris to the poet Stesichorus, citing along the way the commentaries of contemporary humanists, including the celebrated fifteenth-century Florentine humanist Angelo Poliziano.[38] Another physician character, "Martini," intervenes to inquire about Christian sources on blindness and, more pressingly, about what has actually happened to poor Massa, but "Apollonio" has not finished with his excursus on his pagan (and largely Homeric) material, which leads him to cases of virtuous blind men from more recent periods in the history of Greece and Rome.[39] These excurses made no contribution to explaining why Massa had lost his sight; they were very useful, however, as proof of the literary credentials that this circle of physicians possessed.

The multiple voices inherent in the genre of the dialogue allow the author to experiment with diverse viewpoints; Luisin took full advantage of this as well.[40] The general subject of blindness and Massa's particular affliction were grave matters, and Luisin's speakers remain somber as they discuss them. Still, the friends indulge in occasional jokes as their conversation ranges over topics, sometimes in the mode of *serio ludere,* schooling readers while entertaining them. In addition to teasing Massa about his remarkable longevity and playing on the long-standing competition between lawyers and physicians, Luisin's characters pause for a lighthearted debate about whether or not "Christian" and "physician" are antonyms, another trope of literary humanists' invectives against the medical profession. This debate soon becomes an apologia, again by "Apollonio," on the ethics and unassailable Christian credentials of medicine. Putting that particular speech in the mouth of this character was logical insofar as the real Apollonio Massa was a physician. Yet there was perhaps also a measure of irony, or even defense, given Apollonio's tangency to if not membership in the Lutheran world.[41] In a historical moment when thousands of aspiring physicians from northern Europe came to Padua or Bologna, Apollonio Massa had gone to Wittenberg.

Establishing the literary bravura and model Christianity of the medical profession prepared the ground for the arrival of "Nicolò Massa," who appears in the role on which his namesake never ceased to insist: the indefatigable man of letters. When asked if he finds intense study, always difficult and tiring, even more so now that he cannot read on his own, "Massa" insists that this is not the case. If anything, he tells his would-be consolers, who now recede into passive student roles, philosophical studies have become proportionally sweeter as his physical trials have intensified. "I don't recall ever having felt fatigued while studying," he explains, "on the contrary, the pleasure I take in study is infinite."[42]

His Stoic equanimity established, "Massa" does concede that his infirmity requires that he seek assistance, a subject that creates the opportunity for Luisin to move from honoring his colleague as an individual to emphasizing the cultural assets of Massa's family. "I get help with substantial writing and reading," the old man explains, "from my grandson Francesco Grifalconi here, who more than suffices me in these activities, being as capable as he is. But because he obviously cannot attend me every day, needing to leave the house on various business of his own, I have hired a *letterato* who reads aloud the things that I enjoy and writes down what I dictate."[43]

Luisin emphasizes exceptional dedication to humanistic endeavor. We see a physician as devoted to the life of the mind in his eighties—and blind—as he ever was. The talented grandson exemplifies both filial piety and the next generation of literary credentials. We see throughout this dialogue exemplification of the reality, sometimes surprising to modern readers, that philosophy in its ancient and early-modern forms was less a discrete set of ideas to be theorized and more a composite of precepts to be lived.[44] In this portrait ostensibly taken from life, Luisin conveyed distillations of intellectual passion and Stoic equanimity.

In the end, the *Dialogue Entitled Blindness* glorified most the sustaining and illuminating power of literature. Luisin specifies that "Massa" has hired a *letterato,* someone with interdisciplinary competencies and clearly not a medical protégé, to serve him when his grandson cannot be present. This *letterato,* moreover, not only takes dictation, which might involve any subject matter, but also fulfills the craving for pleasure reading. Then as now, reading done for enjoyment (the verb Luisin uses here is *aggradare*) would be literature and not technical material. When pondering the pain and indignities of aging, moreover, "Massa" draws inspiration not from a scientific understanding of bodily decay or even a spiritual reflection on the life to come but instead from meditating on the roster of productive old men from antiquity. None of these examples are physicians. Instead, he confesses, "[I think of] Isocrates the Athenian rhetorician, who at my age dedicated himself to composing the most beautiful oration that he ever wrote, at least among all those one can read now, and that's the *Panathenaicus.* Sophocles and Plato, moreover, exhausted themselves in writing and reading right up to their final hours."[45] Reference to the *Panathenaicus* furnishes a Hellenistic ornamental touch to the ennobling literary-philosophical framework that Luisin sets around the physician "Massa" and, by extension, around the medical profession. In presenting his colleague as the paradigmatic physician-humanist, Luisin followed the rhetorical pattern Massa himself adopted in his self-presentation and in his construction of the medical art. In so doing, Luisin and Massa also followed the preferred style obtaining in the College at large.

Collegiates working in print to enhance the literary dimension of their individual and collective images received models for that undertaking in the course of their regular convocations. Nancy Sirasi has deftly analyzed many relics of the medical community's self-canonization, including academic and funerary orations, which publicized the image of the physician humanist in a pan-European context.[46] One striking example of this phenomenon unearthed in my own research comes from Venice in the year 1563, when Domenico Castelli gave a rousing funeral oration for Vettore

Trincavella, the most illustrious member of the Venetian College of Physicians. According to contemporary reports, a full roster of the College's membership filled the church, together with a crowd of Venetian citizens and even patricians. As one of Trincavella's 155 students, Castelli offered the traditional Latin eulogy.[47]

The breadth of Trincavella's learning constitutes the oration's theme, and we witness each step of Trincavella's precocious genius as he made his way through the academic *cursus honorum*. Castelli explains that he chose to emphasize this theme instead of genteel birth, wealth, or physical prowess not because Trincavella lacked any of these things but because they are comparatively common assets. By contrast, Trincavella's rare genius and intellectual attainments—his unimpeachable cultural legitimacy—deserved commemoration.

Castelli's oration is humanistic hagiography. He presents Trincavella as a selfless man overburdened with intellectual gifts. We see Trincavella at university, making swift progress in rhetoric, dialectic, Greek, and Latin.[48] We learn of Trincavella's growing dedication to medical inquiry as well, but Castelli keeps returning to his subject's breath of expertise and intellectual passion. Even after his reputation as an expert physician and theologian was well established, Trincavella avoided the ire of the "Muses" (poetry and literature) by attending to literary matters even as he worked at mathematics and much else: "While he read the Poets and Historians with the greatest pleasure, he also kept the great works of Geometry and Arithmetic, Music and Astrology often in his hands. He was a man who delighted most in reading many things at the same time, as if indeed he thought thereby to draw around himself a full circle of all the disciplines."[49] Careful to note Trincavella's contributions to "medical humanism," crediting him with helping to correct longstanding corruptions in Galen through his study of the extant Latin and Greek translations of the Arabic commentators and in the light of his own medical practice, Castelli still makes Trincavella's crowning achievement a consequence of his humanistic fervor rather than his medical competence. Trincavella healed princes of all lands and reaped rewards for his services, his encomiast insists, but he had no desire to rest on his laurels. Instead, Trincavella devoted what little leisure time he had to cultivating the liberal arts in the service of the common good: He gave freely to others the knowledge that he had acquired through his exertions.[50] Although Trincavella died a rich man, nonetheless his labors in practical and theoretical medicine connected him to a professional world in which, as our humanistic testators so often stated, exertion still constituted a defining virtue.

Mourners thus received (or endured) a detailed explication of the interdisciplinary cultural ideal that they were expected to emulate. Trincavella offered them a paradigm of the physician-humanist, at once a successful physician, a competent philosopher, and an ardent man of letters. A youth's precocious talent in time extended to all forms of knowledge, which the mature man then generously bequeathed to contemporaries and to posterity as a teacher and author.

Castelli's colleagues listened. Alberto Rini was physically among the attendees; we find a note in his journal that "His Excellency, messer Victor Trincavella, physician and my colleague (who held a lectureship in practical medicine at Padua) was buried . . . and messer Domenico de Castelli gave the oration on Sunday."[51] Rini was in good company. While the College's records strain credulity in claiming that all members were present on this occasion, Trincavella's profile in the medical community had few rivals. And in any case there were fines for absence without excuse at such an event. Further evidence of listening is that Castelli's narrative appeared almost without alteration in Lorenzo Marucini's *vita* of Trincavella, which comprised part of the prefatory material in the posthumous edition of Trincavella's *Opera omnia.*[52]

A collegiate funeral such as Trincavella's emphasized shared commitments, but we might extend their significance beyond the tendency of these occasions to serve as opportunities for celebrating accepted values. Funerary lessons like Castelli's goaded physicians to visit Parnassus no less than anatomical theaters or apothecary shops, to build interdisciplinary libraries, to think of themselves as humanists more than specialists. These encouragements to enhance their cultural legitimacy surely influenced medical doctors' book-buying habits and their consistent practice of testamentary humanism. Medical doctors might well have devised for themselves the image of the physician-humanist, quite apart from the pressures implicit in orations such as Castelli's. Still, those pressures encouraged physicians to express their personal aims in conversation with (if not in dogged conformity to) the recognized ideals of their community and culture.

Members of the Venetian College of Physicians sought myriad ways to prove their humanistic credibility. In the world of print, physicians such as Trincavella emended the classical medical canon. Massa and others, notably Vesalius, offered practical manuals that nonetheless also displayed broad erudition in prefaces and margins. Others, for instance, Fabio Glissenti and Alvise Luisin, positioned themselves explicitly as moral philosophers. Still others published histories and poetry, for example, Lorenzo Marucini. But even those who did not seek out publishing careers also made their own case for medicine as a liberal art in their book bequests and in the breadth of the libraries they collected. As Nancy Siraisi has pointed out, "the strong competitive or performative element in academic life" served as one impetus for physicians to display humanist stripes by diversifying their publications, or at least giving literary, broadly philosophical, or historical learning a good airing in the prefatory material.[53] Yet we must keep in mind that this competitiveness had both positive and negative goals: on the one hand, entering a contest of intellectual virtuosity more or less for its own sake, on the other, contesting a long line of writers who had cast aspersions on the medical profession. Members of the Venetian College of Physicians entered those contests, and even those who did not do so in print reached in their own ways for literary cachet.

MASSA'S BOOKS, COLLEGIATE LIBRARIES

Seeking cultural legitimacy required at minimum some familiarity with literary topics, authors, and texts current in humanistic society. That familiarity, in turn, necessitated hearing about, borrowing, or ideally owning a range of literature. We cannot know the complete contents of Nicolò Massa's library; no full inventory survives. But other family papers attest to a collection of more than one hundred volumes, a size that meshes well with the range of other physicians' collections we have encountered (forty-three to five hundred volumes) and with the fact that nearly half of the physicians represented in book inventory records owned more than one hundred books. In building a picture of the library that Massa amassed and the ways in which it intersects with the humanistic self-conceptions that he and his profession highlighted, we first examine his own remarks about the collection from his testaments, as well as his and his daughter's other papers; then we can examine the rare itemized book inventories of two of his immediate colleagues, Alberto Quattrocchi and Alberto Rini, to suggest the subjects and volumes he might also have acquired.

Massa said a great deal about his library in the course of creating his final will and testament, an enterprise that had many phases from draft to notarization and which occupied him for decades. In an initial twenty-four-folio draft of his will (to which we will return), Massa sketched the contours of a library that certainly served his profession, as he bequeathed medical books to protégés in his line of work, including Francesco Grataruol, but also contained volumes in Italian, Latin, and Greek treating "every sort of science and art."[54] He spent much of this composition attempting to secure this cultural legacy, always described in terms indicating both depth and breadth.

The suggestion of a rich and varied library receives additional confirmation in the household inventory of Massa's principal beneficiary and executor, his daughter Maria Grifalconi, who had been born out of wedlock but whom he had cherished, married to a minor patrician, welcomed home again after she entered widowhood, and treated in every way as his legitimate heir. This inventory notes a large trunk containing seventy-five "printed books of various kinds" (an indication of diverse subject matter) and another "half trunk" that was "full of printed books and manuscripts, both small and large."[55] The books that Grifalconi had come to own would most likely have been outside the realm of medicine. There was no reason for her not to fulfill her father's wish that she give Zuanne Grataruol a portion of the medical books and offer Apollonio Massa borrowing privileges with respect to his other volumes in the field medicine. While other documents in the family archive reveal that she and Apollonio did not get along in later years, there would have been no logical reason to withhold medical books. Her son had entered the law, and, in any case, he died shortly before his grandfather. Given the likelihood, then, that most if not all the medical texts made their way into the libraries of Grataruol and Apollonio Massa, the volumes that remained would have pertained to other subjects. This remainder still constituted a large library by the standards of the day: We have the seventy-five books designated as "various subjects" and at least twenty printed books and manuscripts would have fit into the half-size trunk.

One booklet of household expenditures in Massa's own hand spanning the years 1563 to 1568 teaches us more about his collecting practices.[56] Among quotidian purchases, we find him loaning books to friends and colleagues, which specify some of his bibliographic treasures, as well as elucidating his friendship networks. Massa loaned a collection of Galen's sayings to a physician named Lazaro Fero. He also loaned a copy of Mathiolus's famous herbal to a certain Alvise, son of a barber-surgeon. Massa loaned a book on the art of bathing, possibly the famous work by his colleague Gerolemo Mercuriale, to "His Magnificence, messer Marc'Antonio Novello, Secretary" and his (prohibited) two-volume folio edition of the writings of the theologian Origen (185–254 CE) to his nephew Lorenzo.[57] A "messer Bernardin," son of Zacharia dai Palmagi, borrowed Massa's copy of Leon Battista Alberti's work on human proportions.[58] It makes sense, given these predominantly collegiate networks, that the volumes specified would center on medicine and the human body, but what about the "books of various kinds" that Maria Grifalconi inherited?

To imagine Massa's library, we can take as models the detailed inventories left by two of his immediate colleagues, Alberto Quattrocchi and Alberto Rini. Both these physicians accumulated diverse libraries that made their own sort of case for medicine as a liberal art, showing their owners' dedication to encircling themselves, like Trincavella, with all the disciplines. In so doing Quattrocchi and Rini, like many others at society's middle, satisfied their curiosities and other individual motivations while, from a social perspective, also removing some of the taint of mercenary earning with the astringent of worthy pursuits.

Alberto Quattrocchi's inventory showcases the library of a man with optimal levels of cultural credibility. The assessors called by the Giudici di Petizion on September 12, 1624, to Quattrocchi's household found in his study 339 books ranging across the genres of medicine and literature, across the ancient and modern worlds, across the media of manuscript and print, parchment and paper, folio and octavo.[59] Quattrocchi collected in accordance with some aesthetic and curatorial standards. The assessors found no books in the most affordable duodecimo or seidicesimo editions in his home. And Quattrocchi had probably considered the "statement" that his library would make; he had owned the fifteenth-century Florentine humanist Lorenzo Valla's invective against physicians, which rehearsed the usual criticisms leveled at the medical profession by literary humanists.

Valla would have had to give Alberto Quattrocchi a good deal of credit, had he lived to see this inventory. Roughly half of Quattrocchi's volumes related to medicine, but the rest were humanistic. The most valuable folio editions encompassed the luminaries of the medical canon—Hippocrates, Galen (in a seven-volume set), and Avicenna—and works by illustrious Renaissance physicians Tommaso del Garbo, Girolamo Cardano, Matteus Sylvaticus, and Andreas Vesalius. He also owned loosely related texts by ancient mathematicians and natural philosophers, including Archimedes, Ptolemy, Euclid, and Pliny. But Quattrocchi's library boasted myriad volumes of ancient literature unrelated to medicine. To name just a few, Quattrocchi had invested in folio editions of Livy, Virgil, and Ovid (the *Metamorphoses*). Also in folio we find a Greek lexicon, a Greek dictionary, an anthology of Greek poetry, and two histories of Venice. Nor did Quattrocchi ignore religious writing. His collection of luxury editions also encompassed Boethius, Saint Thomas Aquinas, and several compendia of saints' lives.

The same diverse interests informed Quattrocchi's acquisition of quarto and octavo editions. These volumes appear in far greater numbers than his folio editions, no doubt reflecting their relative affordability. Quattrocchi was attentive to contemporary research on plague and pharmacology, as well as fevers, gynecology, old age, and general medical theory. Interspersed in Quattrocchi's medical collection we even find Prospero Alpini's discourses on Egyptian medicine. But these contributions to his professional library shared shelf space with equal measures of classical literature and contemporary poetry. Quattrocchi also invested in numerous reference materials.[60] He owned a compendium of Paduan legal statutes, a concordance of weights and measures, and a recently published book entitled *Il mercante arrichito,* the sixteenth-century equivalent of "How to Get Rich Quickly." He had also purchased dozens of the self-help manuals then available on the art of memory, including Johann Romberch's *Congestorium artificiose memoriae.*[61] Quattrocchi's reference collection also encompassed Greek-Italian and Spanish-Italian dictionaries and lexicons. Apparently he did not need a Latin dictionary. In another popular category of ready-reference, we find that he also indulged in compilations of *sententiae* (the Renaissance answer to Roget's *Book of Familiar Quotations*), from the classics and the Bible. Quattrocchi also kept current with drama. He owned, for instance, the comedies of the Venetian playwright Andrea Balocco ("Il Ruzzante"). The blending of genres, integration of Latin and vernacular media, and inclusion of numerous self-help manuals in Quattrocchi's library makes his case stand as yet another challenge to binaries of "lay" versus "learned" or "low" versus "high" culture.

Quattrocchi also accumulated titles, authors, and subjects that had appeared on the Index of Prohibited Books. His prohibited collection includes a copy of the Swiss physician-humanist and botanist Conrad von Gesner's *Bibliotheca universalis,* an encyclopedia of all works then known in Latin, Greek, and Hebrew. As Paul Grendler has shown, Gesner's *Bibliotheca* was a favorite among Paduan medical professors with Lutheran tastes.[62] Quattrocchi may have had such a taste. He may also have perused Gesner with an eye to Jewish learning, as he owned several works in this category, including the *Aphorisms* of Rabbi Moses ben Maimon (Maimonides). But of course his Vesalius, too, was prohibited, as were all his astrological books and much of his poetry. Quattrocchi knew the rules, but he ignored them—possibly with relish. He shelved the latest edition of the Index of Prohibited Books next to Gesner's *Bibliotheca.* Indeed, Quattrocchi may even have used the Index in conjunction with Gesner as a buying guide, as Peter Burke has suggested other collectors did.[63]

Such a collection of literature underscores both the diversity of this physician's tastes and his desire to partake of the works most current in humanistic culture. He owned a vernacular translation of Plato, Polybius, a manuscript copy of Cicero's *Letteres familiares.* The latter volume constituted not only a touchstone for card-carrying humanists but also a best seller of the Renaissance enjoying hundreds of print editions in Latin and vernacular translation alike. Yet Quattrocchi signaled the high value he put on his "commerce with the classics" (to borrow Anthony Grafton's evocative phrase) by conducting that exchange in a collector's edition manuscript rather than a demotic print redaction.[64] Another signal of his participation in humanistic culture, Quattrocchi had diverse holdings in Greek history and literature that embraced Herodotus and Thucydides (both in Italian translation), Aesop, Sallust, Porphyry, and Valerius Maximus. His holdings in modern humanist writing included authors from the fifteenth-century, for instance, Pomponio Leto and Angelo Poliziano, up to the latest edition of his fellow citizen Niccolò Doglioni's *Theatro universale,* together with all forms of modern poetry.

No doubt Quattrocchi made some distinctive selections, but overall he formed a collection that would have interested most of his colleagues and the contemporary reading public. Directly akin to the humanist physicians that Nancy Sirasi has unearthed, as well as educated society at large, Quattrocchi devoured history above all. His library included everything from local histories of Venice to universal "histories of the world." Further testament to this historical cosmopolitanism, Quattrocchi owned a history of France (in Latin), an account of the wars of Attila, several accounts of the Ottomans, and Giovanni Antonio Menavino's cultural history of the Turks and Islamic law. Evidently Quattrocchi shared humanists' fascination, masterfully recovered for us by Margaret Meserve, with the Islamic world and in particular the Ottoman Empire.[65] Like the greater part of the reading public in Renaissance Italy, moreover, Quattrocchi had a penchant for biography, itself a branch of history as well as philosophy teaching by example.[66] He preferred the exploits of famous military men in antiquity, but his compendia of saints' lives and martyrologies prove that he also attended to exemplary lives in the Christian context.

Other physicians proved, like Quattrocchi, to be literary omnivores, reinforcing the notion that these records help us form an accurate general picture of the library of Nicolò Massa and other members of this milieu. Alberto Rini, for instance, found himself the beneficiary of the libraries of both his physician father and lawyer brother. The 1604 inventory of his bibliographic inheritance, plus his own additions, reveals a library that had grown to five hundred volumes.[67] We might expect this collection to be even more weighted toward medicine than Quattrocchi's, given that three of the four collectors were physicians. Yet the Rini medical library shows even more diversity. Counting any ancient or modern texts directly useful for practical medicine, the "professional library" constitutes only 4 percent of the collection. To be sure, the Rini family owned copies of Aristotle and Galen, with commentaries, as well as recent contributions by their brethren, including Gerolemo Mercuriale's *De arte gymnastica,* Gerolemo Fracastoro's complete works (including his epic poem on syphilis), Castore Durante's *The Treasure of Health,* and an astonishingly beautiful illustrated herbal (in manuscript) bequeathed to Alberto by his father, Benedetto. But the Rini library gave pride of place to genres outside medicine.

The categories that dominated the Rini family's interests paralleled Quattrocchi's literary collection. Here, too, we find an array of ancient authors and contemporary humanist writing (especially history), as well as theology and devotional literature. Books in the liberal arts constituted 58 percent of this collection. Together, medicine and the other sciences (especially astronomy and astrology) comprise only 6 percent. And, despite the fact that one donor was a lawyer, only 9 percent of the books pertain specifically to legal practice. Even these professional men, then, collected less like specialists and more like generalists. Or perhaps it would be better to say they curated more like generalists. We have witnessed many testators bequeathing books related to their professions to men in the same line of work; so, we may safely assume that the light representation of medical books in physicians' inventories reflects, at least in part, the prior dispersal of volumes on medicine to colleagues and students. All the same, that a professional family kept intact its literary materials more than its occupational ones indicates that general literature held an importance similar to other jealously guarded assets. Like real estate or other valuables, humanistic literature was not to be dispersed but transmitted intact. If financial patrimony promised to sustain the family at a pragmatic level, literature served as tangible evidence of its cultural legitimacy.

In the case of the Rini library, the reputation for broad learning he enjoyed while alive brought many borrowers to his door. Book seekers came to Rini for anything but medical texts. At the end of one of his remarkable account books (which we examine in detail in Chapter 5), he lists all the books that he had recently loaned to friends and colleagues. This list mirrors the diversity of Quattrocchi's library. The most notable genre that friends sought was history: old chronicles and modern historical narratives; Contarini's history of the Italian Wars and the histories of Paolo Giovio, who also a physician by profession; Bartoli's history of Venice and a general history of Spain. But Rini had other forms of humanist writing to offer as well. A friend hungry for poetry got from him Sabellico's sonnets. Others, perhaps interested in the ancient traditions connected with the contemporary Ottoman world, borrowed a narrative of Emperor Alexander's Persian campaigns.[68] A similar list of loans appears toward the end of Rini's second journal and again displays a predominance of history (for instance, Pietro Bembo's *History of Venice* and Bonaldi's chronicles) and poetry, especially the *Rime* of Torquato Tasso. We also find works of biography, epistles, and sermons. Rini also loaned out two biographical accounts of the Barbaro family, a collection of epistles by Mantuan humanists, and the sermons of Francesco Panigarola, a Franciscan friar and prolific author of sermons and treatises on the art of memory.[69]

But we might wonder what the Rini library could tell us about a physician's tastes. After all, several members of the family contributed, and we might expect them to favor different subjects. Fortunately, Rini's own account books also detail the volumes he bought for himself and these underscore the precedence of literature that the Rini library as a whole displays. Over the course of twenty-two years (1576–1598), Rini's journals note the purchase of seventy-two individual volumes, for sixty of which Rini provided the name of the author and sometimes also the title and publisher. Perhaps aware that he had an increasingly limited time for completing the collection that would embody his own intellectual passions, Rini became an especially avid book-hunter in the last five years of his life. Rini purchased fewer than ten books between the years 1576 and 1580 and only six between 1581 and 1586. By contrast, he bought twenty books between 1587 and 1592 and nearly forty between 1593 and 1598. The bookshops most often furnished him with ancient literature, history, and biography. The liberal arts trumped all Rini's other interests, comprising 57 percent of the books he amassed. By contrast, only 30 percent of Rini's purchases concerned theology or devotion, and only 13 percent of the acquisitions he made in two decades can be classified as medical or scientific texts.[70] In other words, Rini bought like a humanist.

Members of Venice's College of Physicians who flourished in the latter part of the sixteenth century display a bibliophilia that simply does not fit within the interpretive model of the "professional" library. Fifteenth-century Venetian physicians do seem to have collected most intensely in their occupational fields.[71] And even in sixteenth-century France, physicians still accumulated books directly pertinent to their medical work.[72] But Venetian physicians of the sixteenth century cherished literature, suggesting both dissemination of humanistic fervor outside the ranks of that movement's leadership and the pressures of contemporary humanistic ideals on urban professionals. We know that in the early-modern period generalists earned more praise than specialists did. Collegiate physicians exerted themselves in seeking and appropriating that broad knowledge. Desire no doubt provided one motive, but confronting prejudices offered another.

Confidence in the power of letters to secure cultural legitimacy characterizes the print publications that Massa and his colleagues authored. Physicians also furnished proof of their cultivation in the large and diverse libraries they accumulated. The hopes that Massa and his colleagues cherished for their cultural work, however, emerge best in their testaments.

LITERARY LEGACIES

While publications afford the most direct access to the ideas and personae that our subjects crafted for consumption, the archives are not silent on matter of their minds. Considering the Massa family papers, Richard Palmer rightly points out that they "reveal only a little about Massa's intellectual interests and medical practice."[73] Thus Palmer focused most on the economic story that these documents tell, as they were intended to do. But although comparatively laconic about cultural matters, the Massa papers nonetheless repay examination for the "little" they reveal about the family's intellectual and literary priorities. Here, too, we find evidence of Massa's insistence on the themes of autonomy and self-invention, including his self-conception as a man of letters. And the pride Massa derived from being the head of an intellectual family is more evident here than in the formal works he authored.

By far the most discursive of the Massa private family documents is his autograph draft will of 1562, which covers twenty-four folios (roughly fifty double-spaced typed pages in our world).[74] Naturally, as this was a draft, part of its length derives from Massa's edits and reiterations as he sought the most unassailable language in which to articulate his final wishes. Complexities of financial and real estate transactions, precisely the matters that Palmer analyzed, also loom large in this document. Yet intellectual matters also figured in Massa's complex calculus of family, property, and an honorable legacy.

Massa began his draft will with a paragraph of legal boilerplate in Latin, as notaries did, but reworked this moment of Latinity in ways that infused the statement with more cultural meaning than any notary would have done. Minus particulars of parentage, neighborhood, and occupation, the formula for commencing a final testament in the late Renaissance was some version of this very straightforward statement: "In the name of God Eternal, I, sound in mind, realizing that death is common to all but the hour it will strike unpredictable, have deemed it prudent to arrange my affairs now. Accordingly, I have called upon the notary hereafter indicated to write/validate this, my final will and testament." By contrast, Massa begins: "You, God and Father Omnipotent, and Jesus Christ Your Son, and the Holy Spirit, One Eternal God, I supplicate you with my whole heart, beseeching and praying that you enlighten my mind, and govern it, lest I should write anything unjust or beside the point, or introduce material that could give anyone a pretext for litigation, in this my final testament and final will. And I will now begin to write this testament in the vernacular, so as to make it more readily understood."[75]

At one level, Massa aligns himself with Catholic Reformation piety, attenuating his expression of the standard invocation "in the name of God Eternal" to emphasize his orthodox conception of the Trinity.[76] But Massa also used his Latin phrasing, complete with subjunctive clauses of negative purpose, to underscore his status as a man of learning. There was no need, moreover, for a testator to explain why they had decided to write the introduction of their will in Latin and the rest in Italian; this was standard practice by the mid-sixteenth century. The Latin framing represented the document's legal authority while the Italian body text maximized comprehension. That Massa felt compelled to prove that he could express himself in Latin, but chose not to do so at length in the interest of (lesser) readers' comprehension, indicates his desire to flaunt his linguistic abilities. Indeed, Massa shared this desire with two of his colleagues, Valerio Superchio and Francesco Longo, who offered similar superfluous explanations in their wills. "Even though I am a professor of letters," Superchio troubled to specify, "I have written this in the vernacular in the interest of serving the better comprehension of those who will have to read and execute it."[77] After all we have seen of physicians' bids for cultural credibility, it is perhaps not astonishing to find these indications of intellectual pride even in a textual space designated for humbling oneself before God.

Disposition of properties, no less than souls, occupied all testators, Massa among them. Yet this physician had particular cultural concerns relating to his literary and bibliographic legacies. Part of his anxiety derived from the fact that his chosen heir and executor, his daughter Maria Grifalcone, had been born both female and illegitimate. Grifalcone's double vulnerability by extension endangered his estate and necessitated giving her strong legal protections. Massa not only deployed the usual phrases against litigation arising from the greed of untrustworthy family members; he also tapped male relatives and associates to assist her. Massa had legally recognized and legitimized his daughter, but he feared (rightly) that these formalities would do her little good if court battles arose. Time and again, he struggles to find the strongest language for marking Maria as his heir and forbidding that at any time "anyone at all, whosoever they might be" *(mai alcuno, et sia chi esser si voglia)* could challenge or inconvenience her. Massa felt a paternal desire to save his child from trouble, but at the same time he sought to protect his cultural legitimacy; he had vested his literary no less than his biological patrimony in Maria Grifalcone.

Massa bequeathed to his daughter the stewardship of his library, together with her choice of all books in Latin and Italian that she should wish for her own use. He also gave her the full contents of his *studio.* Given Massa had male students and male relatives with university degrees and careers, bestowing his cultural estate on his daughter might have struck contemporaries as strange, if not actionable. What might have prompted this choice—especially puzzling, given the potential difficulties that her (natal) illegitimacy might pose? Part of the answer relates to humanistic practices, which included appointment of daughters as literary heirs to their fathers.[78] In humanist circles, fathers derived considerable cultural capital from having a learned daughter, since the father–daughter intellectual pairing was one of the many relational models that Italian humanists borrowed from ancient literary luminaries, paradigmatically Hortensius and Cicero. While Massa displays great fondness for his daughter and the utmost trust in her judgment, he may also have borrowed this notion of a daughterly simulacrum for his intellectual ideals, as he did so much else, from the humanists.

What objects beyond books did the young widow stand to inherit? "I find myself in possession of various kinds of moveable goods," Massa explains, "among which there are works of silver and gold, jewels, rings, coins, tapestries, and other assorted household ornaments, as well as books and other things of mine that I will not list individually."[79] One of the rings received specific characterization as a cameo ring of reputedly ancient provenance. He described the object as "a little gold ring set with a carnelian on which are engraved some figures on horseback and others standing—and it's believed to be an ancient engraving."[80] Evidently Massa, like many people of humanistic aspiration, collected art objects and antiquities.[81] At all events, unsatisfied with his description of his wishes with regard to the *studio,* he returns at several points to rework this clause. "I leave to the aforementioned Maria all my movable goods that are found in my house or outside my house in whatever place you will," he expresses it late in the draft, "and of whatever sort you can imagine, included in which I mean to indicate gold and silver, rings, jewels, and every other sort of ornament for the studies, or rooms," a locution he straightaway changes to "[movable goods] of the house that may be found, both in the rooms and in the studies and in my trunks of all sorts."[82] That he tested several different versions of this passage indicates a preoccupation with his cultural estate of nearly the same magnitude as that concerning his real estate.

The issues of books and learning return with force when Massa considers his nephews and grandson. As of 1562, Massa had only harsh words for Apollonio (this would change in time), viewing this nephew and protégé as the worst of ingrates. In a sentence that would have tested even Cicero's forbearance, Massa castigates his protégé in ways that help us understand the central place he accorded advanced education in his conception of family honor:

> I leave to the aforementioned Apollonio, whom I have kept in my house from the time when he was in swaddling bands to the moment he wanted to marry madonna Gratiosa, daughter of the late nobleman messer Lorenzo di Martini (the lawyer), and whom I have fed, raised, and made to continue his education at various institutions of higher learning, and made him a doctor of arts and medicine, for all of which I have spent every cent of my not inconsiderable income, in addition to the many efforts I have made on his behalf, and many headaches and troubles I've had on his account, of this my money that I have spent for him, and given to him at various times, some of which I have noted in my account books and many I have not, and the ones I have not noted are far more numerous than those which I have recorded, of the many monies given to him and by him spent, as partly one can see in the letters he wrote to me in which he mentioned having received them, and also in the letters in which he begged me to be willing to send him money, and also in the letters of exchange paid out for him, and other expenses made at other times, of all of which he is debtor to me, all that debt of his, and my credit, of monies loaned to him as of expenses and payments made for him I bequeath to him by way of an inheritance and as fulfillment of any claim that he could conceivably believe he has owing to him from me, through any means whatsoever.[83]

At one level, we see a caregiver's traditional complaint about sums of money, time, and energy lavished on a sometimes prodigal and perhaps insufficiently grateful relation. Massa also offers us a testament to the importance of education and merit in his conception of family responsibility, which connects to his own sense of intellectual agency and honor. The familial and the personal intertwine in fascinating ways. Massa even retains the subject position as he describes Apollonio's progress through the academic course of honors: "I made him study at various schools and universities" *(io lo [l'ho] . . . fato studiar in diversi studi)* and "I made him become a doctor of arts and medicine" *(et fatosi dottor delle Arte et medicine).* This physician strongly supported his nephew's studies, but freighted those benefactions with the highest expectations. And his very insistence on the wearying nature of the efforts he expended in educating this ingrate monumentalized his paternalistic virtues.

In arranging the bequest for his other nephew, Lorenzo, another orphaned dependent, Massa speaks again of tireless devotion to the academic progress of a young relation. Yet here, in speaking of Lorenzo, Massa adopts a more avuncular tone and exhibits more generosity. While the bulk of Lorenzo's bequest, like Apollonio's, consisted not of new gifts but the cancellation of debt for educational expenses and cash loans during his years of study, Massa at least gives this nephew credit for making a good cultural return on his uncle's capital investment. Here Massa describes with satisfaction that his money and effort had ensured "that [Lorenzo] learned both good comportment and the humanities here in the city, in Padua and elsewhere, such that he might become a man honored on account of his own virtues, as he has in fact become."[84] The subject position in this statement wavers in a telling way. While Massa still takes credit for seeing to it that Lorenzo had the benefit of a humanistic education, Lorenzo's later enhancements to the family's intellectual honor warranted recognition on their own merits. For Massa, the highest virtue was self-determination, earning honor for one's own accomplishments, and especially doing so within the field of culture. But we should also bear in mind that, as we have seen, physicians no less than any other men tended to expect one son to follow them in their occupation but aimed to situate others at a higher level; in the case of medical men, a common goal was to get one son into the law. Massa may thus have categorized Apollonio's achievements as the minimum requirement to maintain the family's professional reputation. Lorenzo's work in "good letters," by contrast, enhanced his family's cultural legitimacy.

Looking further into his family's cultural future, Massa positions his daughter and, through her, ultimately his grandson Francesco as his intellectual heirs—even despite the care lavished on his successful nephews. These considerations return us once again to Massa's library. This patriarch entrusted his lettered daughter to loan his nephews volumes at her discretion, but insisted that at no time should she feel constrained to make loans. He also enjoined her to keep careful note of any books she had decided to loan to her cousins and recall them instantly if ever Francesco, any other child she might have, or she herself needed them. He even troubles to state that while Apollonio might wish to consult some of the medical books, Maria should nonetheless retain full power to reclaim even these technical texts "if she needs them back, either for herself or for her children" and that she should do with these books as with all the others "precisely as seems best to her."[85] Massa could not have made a clearer statement of his intention to keep his bibliographic legacy safely under the control of his designated heir and her descendants.

Massa's consideration of books leads directly to planning Francesco's upbringing and education. At the time of this will, Francesco was approximately thirteen years old, and his preparatory studies would have been close to concluding and thoughts of university pressing. Noting that he loved the boy most affectionately and pleading that he had done everything to protect him from the lawsuits and other attacks coming at him from his deceased father's side of the family, Massa then promises not to say anything more about Francesco, who is in the capable hands of an affectionate mother. Like many grandparents, however, he cannot entirely keep that promise. "I won't say anything more," Massa writes, "except that I commend him first to Our Lord God, who is the chief protector of schoolchildren and widows, and next I commend him to Maria his mother, although I'm aware of how very much she loves him, knowing how much toil and inconvenience and hassle she has endured to bring him up properly. And I urge her to continue raising him in the fear and reverence of God and instilling good manners in him, and making him keep going in his profitable studies of the humanities and Christian virtue."[86] Massa envisioned his daughter performing the same pedagogical role for her son that he himself had performed with his nephews. The typology of the parent that we see from Massa was one who would endure remarkable quantities of "expense, hassle, inconvenience" to see to it that youths learned not only Christian virtue and good manners but humanistic letters. Much as his characterization of Lorenzo indicated, Massa conceived of Francesco's training as an essential part of making not only a good person but one who would be honored for his merits.

Massa situates himself as a member of an aspiring middling sort through his powerful faith in the autonomy and range of cultural motion that that humanistic pursuits promised. His reflexive linking of "good manners and habits," Christian virtue, and the humanities in the formation of an honorable reputation merely expresses with more detail what we have seen many other practitioners of testamentary humanism refer to as the formula for "becoming a man" or "becoming a man of the right sort." Massa, too, imagined his male heirs and affines as serving the family best in earning reputations as *uomini da bene*. And much as artisans, merchants, and priests imagined books and education as catalysts for that transformation, so, too, did Massa. Unlike many of these other Venetians, Massa had provided proof of his own cultural legitimacy in his published works. Why the anxieties in his case? Much as we saw with the priest Paulo Pincio, Massa's heir had a stigma to confront. Much like Superchio, moreover, he hoped to see his relations get beyond medicine as such, still suffering a degree of stigmatization as a profession, and into the safer professional terrain of the law. What he set down in this alternative medium, then, were his efforts to ensure the success of a new generation of literati.

In a final will of 1569 Massa streamlined and intensified the testamentary humanism developing in his draft will.[87] These two documents are closely linked; nothing dramatic had changed in his general outlook or tone, save that Apollonio had by this point earned more goodwill from his uncle and that Massa now expressed his bequests with more economy, having worked through his doubts in the earlier draft. Massa's principal beneficiary and executor remained his daughter, now widowed and bereft of her son, who had died earlier that year. Massa's other executors were Apollonio and Lorenzo, together with one of Massa's protégés in the College, Zuanne Grataruol, whom he claimed to love "like a son." While Massa trusts all his executors to make good decisions regarding his estate by democratic voting, he insists that if in any doubt Maria's view constitutes the majority opinion and no action might be taken without her approval.

Most interesting for our purposes, Massa sharpened his already pointed literary bequest in the final iteration of his testament. Given that years, illnesses (even blindness), the death of his grandson, and ongoing disputes with Maria's marital kin had transpired between the time of the draft will and this final version, we might have expected literary matters to move to the margins—if not fall by the wayside. On the contrary, books become even more central. Maria remained her father's principal intellectual heir. Massa leaves her, together with Apollonio and Lorenzo, as executor of his literary estate and library, of which she is to have first pick of any volumes she may desire for her own use. "I leave to the aforementioned Maria my daughter," he explains, "and to messers Apollonio and Lorenzo my nephews, the responsibility of serving as executors of all my books, but first . . . Maria should take out at her own choice whichever of the Latin or vernacular books appeal to her."[88] The importance Massa attached to his literary property is unmistakable here, and he returns to the subject at several points in his testament for good measure.

Massa now asks his nephews to scrutinize his whole library and remove any volumes that may be "prohibited by the Holy Ordinances of the Council [of Trent], or are otherwise against good morals," either burning them or "doing whatever has been established as proper procedure by the Holy Council."[89] Certainly Massa played the role of a good son of the Catholic Reformation. Indeed, he gives us an intriguing litmus test for the intensity of that movement, as he did not include this clause in his draft will, written only seven years previously. In 1562, the Council of Trent was just moving to conclusion; by 1569, evidently its effects were clearly felt even in Venice.[90] But we should be careful about taking Massa's pious injunctions at face value. After all, he had already specified as the first act regarding his library that Maria should take any volumes in Italian or Latin that she pleased. This clause left his heir free to claim the whole library, excepting his Greek books, and she might thereby save many forbidden books in the collection from pious flames. We should not assume, then, that Massa's views aligned with the objectives of the Index.

Having asserted his status both as a learned man and a pious book owner, Massa turns his attention to preserving intact his humanistic collection. He once again instructs his executors to give his protégé, Zuanne Grataruol, any of his texts on practical medicine that Grataruol might find useful.[91] By urging his heirs to make his medical library available to Grataruol, Massa used his professional collection to recognize bonds of professional kinship, but these volumes were in that sense more expendable than those he refused to alienate from his bloodline. In a final passage, Massa considers the remainder of his library. As he turns to his broader, humanistic collection, he speaks in terms not merely of intellectual and professional honor but of the deepest family bond: "As concerns the division of my books, I ordain that my nephews and daughter proceed as follows: if they take books for themselves, they must take the subjects and volumes whole—and not dismember them. And I beseech all three of them to love one another and live together in peace and tenderness, treating each other as siblings, with God's peace and the peace of Jesus Christ."[92] This apparent non sequitur poignantly asserts the significance this old, blind physician attached to his library. Massa moves from forbidding them to pull one volume from a series, or cutting one section from a book ("dismembering" his library), to exhorting them to bind themselves as siblings in Christ's peace. Linking the bindings of books to the bonds of blood, Massa entreated his executors to keep both his literary collection and his family intact. In Massa's view, his own labor had built both his family and his library from nothing.

Nicolò Massa spoke with particular eloquence about letters and his intellectual patrimony, but the basic priorities informing his expressions mesh well with those of his colleagues. Other physicians similarly spoke of the honors they accumulated, the credentials and reputations they developed and the ways in which they hoped these assets would help preserve—and, in some cases, advance—their families. We will consider similar reflections as we turn to Francesco Longo and Alberto Rini in subsequent chapters. But the most useful comparison for present purposes is the testamentary hectoring of Valerio Superchio. If Massa spoke of cultural patrimony in worried elegiac, Superchio did so in obsessive commandments. In both cases, however, the remarks expressed an academic standard for measuring the value of both self and kin.

In his 1540 will, Superchio specified that one older son, Tiberio, was to follow him into the field of medicine, but a younger son, Alessandro, was enjoined to obtain a doctorate in law.[93] Superchio also had five daughters, several of whom he had managed similarly to situate a notch up the social ladder. One daughter, Barbara, married a Captain Antenor di Leonardi; another, Isabetta, married a count from Montelabbate. Superchio notes that he bequeathed to these daughters ten ducats each "as a sign of love," emphasizing that they did not need the money, both of them having married so well that they "live as if they were patrician women [*come se fussero signore*]." Rather, he intended this bequest as a symbolic apology for his inability to provide them with higher dowries years before. "When I arranged the marriages of these two older girls," Superchio explains, "I was culturally rich but cash poor, having no more than seventy ducats to my name."[94] The marriages that Superchio arranged for most of his daughters suggest strategic social advancement. The four bridegrooms were the patrician Zuanne Giacomo di Leonardi, from Pasano, who was also a doctor of laws; the Count of Montelabbate, who, according to Superchio, was as of 1540 "an orator in Venice for the Illustrissimo Signore Aura de Urbino"; Captain Antenor di Leonardi, the brother of the aforementioned Zuanne Giacomo di Leonardi; and "the most excellent Doctor of Arts and Medicine, messer Agustin Bellaro, from Feltre." The youngest daughter had to content herself with the "spettabile" Andrea Piscina, probably a wealthy merchant, notary, or jurist.[95] Two of Superchio's daughters, then, married within his social bracket, one endogamously to a physician, another to some sort of merchant, but two others made patrician matches.

Superchio's pride in his family's social mobility is clear, as is the delight he took in his boastful insistence that his own merit had made all this possible. Like Massa, Superchio viewed himself as a self-made man of letters. He had become a man of cultural standing when he arranged matches for his elder daughters—"ero richo de animo et de honore" (literally, "rich in spirit and honor")—even if impecunious. Superchio suggests that his cachet compensated for his lack of cash. Intellectual credentials, then, could quickly shade into social and financial capital. Superchio, the physician, could boast at the end of his life of having a son who was a lawyer and two married daughters "living as if they were patricians." Superchio would have agreed with Pierre Bourdieu's conception of cultural capital and its uses. Massa would likely have done so as well, to a degree, but his final hope to conserve, not cash in, the bonds between his collection and his kin suggests the limitations of that model, as we move case to case.

At the edge of full membership in the humanist *respublica litterarum*, Nicolò Massa the self-made man of letters at least earned notice from Francesco Sansovino. More practically, he also had an heir who tended his legacy and built him an elegant tomb. Maria Massa Grifalcone indeed preserved much of his library, as her household inventory demonstrated. Lacking a blood heir at the time she wrote her own will, Grifalcone preserved the collection for future generations by donating it to a charitable foundation, along with most everything else she owned. She chose as her principal heir the Zitelle, a women's shelter of sorts, which attended to Venetian girls at risk of falling into sexual service. But this institution had connections to the literary world as well. The contemporary courtesan and poet Veronica Franco had encouraged women to choose a life at the Zitelle in lieu of her own fate, and its directors had a clear mandate to watch out for attractive and well-educated daughters of artisan, merchant, or patrician families who lacked dowries or whose chastity had been (or seemed likely to be) compromised, and who might thus have ended up plying Franco's trade.[96]

As another and more direct service to Nicolò Massa's legacy, Grifalcone also paid the sculptor Alessandro Vittoria two hundred ducats to execute a funerary monument for her father, to which Vittoria would later add a portrait of her cousin Apollonio.[97] These marble monuments constitute the mute relics of this family's cultural legitimacy. Far more lively is its "paper memory," to borrow Matthew Lundin's eloquent term, the thousands of words Massa left in print and manuscript.[98] The same connection between obsessive writing and the anxieties of upward mobility that Lundin found in the contemporary lawyer Hermann Weinsberg seems to have existed for this Venetian physician.[99] The marble bust, then, served not to state but only to underscore Massa's association with a level of social respect among people "of the right sort" for which he and other physicians campaigned vigorously.

Nicolò Massa's aims centered the fortune of his family, but not all physicians looked on their literary learning, collecting, and thinking in such instrumental ways. If Massa and, even more so, the irascible Superchio, directed matters of the mind and letters toward socioprofessional advancement, we also find in the ranks of Venice's College of Physicians different aspirations. We turn now to Francesco Longo, whose ethical wills reveal hopes that had more to do with edification than with social mobility. Longo confronted as many worries as Nicolò Massa did, and he had a background even more ordinary. However, Longo represented his travails not as "hassles and headaches" but instead as crucibles for his moral philosophy.

CHAPTER 4

FRANCESCO LONGO'S PHILOSOPHICAL TESTAMENTS

On March 28, 1574, the physician Francesco Longo summoned a notary to his house in the tiny parish of San Marcilian, at the northwestern edge of the city of Venice. Longo remained sound in body and mind even at the age of sixty-eight—a remarkably good run for the era, as he conceded. It was time to make his final will and testament, always an unpleasant task.[1] Even the most straightforward part of this endeavor, arranging the disposition of his property, raised anxious questions: What if his heirs should fight, as so many did, over their inheritances? How could he be sure that the written word, however carefully chosen, would convey his precise meaning? As a man of learning, he knew that every syllable has a vast semantic range. Longo had taken his first doctorate in the liberal arts at the University of Padua in 1530 and his second in medicine, also at Padua, in 1535.[2] Like most of his colleagues, he could have written this document in his own hand and even in Latin, but he no longer had the strength. Longo had also made a testament twenty-two years previously, during an illness.[3] He knew how to go about the task then, but life had become more difficult in the meantime. And his personality further complicated the undertaking. Like all testators, Longo aimed to put his property in order, but for him "legacy" meant ethical precepts as much as cash or household goods.

Who surrounded the old physician as he embarked on his final testament? The notary Giovanni Girolamo Longin appeared at Longo's sickbed that day, fortunately with ample supplies. Most testators, from tile workers to doges, had little to say. In a few sentences or, at most, a few pages, they bequeathed their property to wives, husbands, and children, leaving perhaps a ducat or two to one of the city's charitable foundations after Longin had prodded them on the point, as Venetian notaries were required by law to do.[4] Longo, however, was that rarer client who took an expansive approach to the testament; he would require not the usual single sheet of paper but almost ten full folios to make his wishes known. Longin's hand would cramp before the job was done. Two other men appeared to serve as witnesses, verifying the speaker's identity and, in due course, attesting that the written text matched the dictation. As usual, the witnesses were colleagues and friends of the testator. In this case, they were Adrian Vidal, a pharmacist who now ran the apothecary shop once owned by Longo's father, Pietro, and Flamino de Ca' de Mezzo, a nobleman whose friendship Longo had made thanks to the ascent along the social ladder that the medical profession initiated.

Since the testament existed as a secret trust between testator, notary, and witnesses until the postmortem publication of the document, these four men became the protagonists of the event.[5] But for Longo, as for many testators, family and friends were present in mind if not the room. By this point in his long life, he had lost many of his closest family members, including his wife, Marietta, who had died nine years earlier, and his younger brother, Girardo, who had passed away long before that, probably in the plague of 1555. Yet many other people remained to be considered in this document. Longo's daughter, Virginia, had taken her vows at the nearby convent of Corpus Domini around 1562, but he continued to look after her. He also had three sons to consider. Pietro, the eldest, had taken his medical degree from the College of Physicians in Venice in 1556 and was now a practicing physician in his own right.[6] Longo's youngest, Nonio Cornelio, had aspirations as an entrepreneur.[7] These two young men would be the old doctor's principal heirs. Giulio, Longo's middle son, elicited fatherly concern but could not be a major beneficiary, because he had suffered an incapacitating ailment or accident.

Francesco Longo had a share of worries equal to those of most testators, but he dictated a will on that March day that modeled Stoic equanimity and emotional equilibrium. Longo's testament is an unusual, but not a unique, document. Like the artisans, merchants, priests, and especially the other physicians we have met, this doctor used his testament to construct a monument of character and learning. He shared with other testamentary humanists the determination to insert claims to cultural legitimacy even within constraints of notarial boilerplate. But Longo chose to make these claims less in fretful passages of self-glorification and more through philosophical lessons.

The pedagogical and ethical qualities of Longo's last thoughts strike the reader from the outset. Early-modern testators, as we have seen, were expected to begin by bequeathing their souls, humbly and with penitence, to God. Longo, like Nicolò Massa and other humanistic testators we have encountered, eventually made that spiritual bequest, but he began with himself and a display of his learning. He made elegant rhetoric and moral reflections out of the usual legal preamble:

> I have often been moved to consider a subject that no one can ever ponder too often and that few people ever consider sufficiently—that is, our end, or death. This train of thought, this meditation, can never be unnecessary, nor can it ever be too carefully pondered. Knowing that death is a certainty for everyone, but our final hour impossible to guess, I have thought it both useful and proper for each person to ponder their affairs before death strikes—death, which forebodes her imminent presence to us through the myriad and various moments of doubt we feel in the midst of our daily business. Yet many people brush aside these warnings, not realizing that death is quite near to them, even though they are young, not in their dotage, as I am, having by God's grace lived sixty-eight years sound in body and in mind. And so I have set out to put in order both myself and my possessions, and wish to organize everything in this my final will—though, to tell the truth, my belongings are so few and so trifling that I am almost ashamed to mention them in a testament. Still, rich and poor alike worry about their possessions, however unequal their estates may be.[8]

Longo thus traced his philosophy, putting himself forward as a model testator and pointing out the dangerous negligence of others. He had already begun dispensing advice to an imagined audience that no doubt included his immediate heirs, Pietro and Nonio Cornelio, but his phrasing and use of the first person plural rather than the second alerts us that he had more than these young men in mind; his vision of audience encompassed posterity in its fullest sense. He declared to himself, his sons, the notary, witnesses, other family, and anyone else who might then or at any time see this stack of paper that "we" must attend to the odd moments of uncertainty in the midst of day-to-day business, as they may be death's reminders that we might leave this world at any moment and urging us to prepare ourselves for that voyage. Longo even paused to reflect on the equality of rich and poor: We all worry about our possessions and legacies. Longo's claim to belong to the ranks of the poor, terming his estate a collection of "trifles," did stretch the truth. He was no land magnate, but his possessions included a residence, two rental apartments, and small plots of land on the *terraferma,* as well as modest investments, including his wife's artisan-level dowry of fifteen hundred ducats. Like many testators, Longo under-valued his possessions to reduce the notarial fees (usually a portion of the total value of the estate) as well as the taxes his heirs would have to pay. Still, on the economic standards of this wealthy city, Longo's financial situation even at a generous estimate put him on the low end of the middling ranks. His textual wealth, by contrast, was considerable. In his own way, Longo's testament would make a statement similar to Valerio Superchio's. Here we have another man who was "cash poor, but culturally rich." Longo displayed even from the outset evidence of his intellectual and literary assets. His first sentences draw out universal meaning from an individual case (himself, as it happened), a characteristic manner of working for a thinker and, given the precepts he derived, a moral philosopher.

Although a man with a clear rhetorical bent, Longo apparently did not publish—at least nothing has yet come to light. And while in relatively comfortable circumstances, Longo's income did not stretch to patronage or elaborate funerary monuments. This testament would become the principal artifact of his honor as a man of experience, learning, and good character. He devised practical instructions and legacies, to be sure, but throughout this document he bequeathed further ethical and philosophical ruminations.

Longo's philosophical final testament together with an earlier will that evinces the same qualities and strategies offer rich opportunities for anatomizing another quest for cultural legitimacy. Longo shared much with colleagues in prioritizing intellectual and literary matters. And as a man who had lived the realities of social mobility, his circumstances no doubt played a role in urging him to prove or emphasize his learning. Yet Longo's wills teach us new things about the sense of meaning and even satisfaction that his encounters with books brought him, which in turn show us the limitations of a purely instrumental vision of cultural legitimacy. Longo cared about status and mobility, but not with the same intensity. He wanted to prove his cultural worth for social reasons, and he wanted posterity to know that he had a university education and books; he also wanted us to see a character that put good learning to good purposes. Longo aligned with the dominant approach to Italian Renaissance philosophy that Christopher Celenza has shown to be a set of objectives derived from the ancient canon aimed at living an ethically exemplary life, rather than a discrete hermeneutic or school of thought—an emphasis on lived practices that had much in common with ancient precedent, as Pierre Hadot has explained.[9] Longo had more tenuous connections to the humanistic world than Massa did. Not only do we have no publications from Longo, he also misquotes his sources in a way that suggests studies not quite as rigorous as Massa's. Yet that relative distance from the intellectual elite may have kindled in Longo, as it did in other testators even more tangential positions, an even more humanistic spirit. *Eruditi* teach us about literary culture, of course, but aspirants (however flawed) reveal its ideals with a force all their own.

LIVING AND DYING WELL: LESSONS FROM A PERSIAN KING

The single greatest concern for Francesco Longo was to unify his heirs. Like many testators, he invoked Christ's peace; unlike many, he did not leave the matter there. For Longo, biblical injunction in itself did not ensure unanimity, a defining value in Venetian civic and moral philosophy, as Margaret King and others have taught us.[10] The image of the requisite power came instead from the first-century Greek biographer, historian, and moral philosopher Plutarch, and specifically from Plutarch's *Moralia.*[11]

The figure Longo chose as the image for his beneficiaries' close contemplation was one that he imagined to be the ancient Persian king Artaxerxes. Longo reminds his sons that he has always wished them to be "of one will and spirit," and that this wish is all the more urgent in light of his impending departure from the world. In this wish and at this moment, he explains, "I have in mind what Artaxerxes, the most famous king of the Persians, did when he was close to death, which was to have a great bundle of spear shafts brought before his sons—a bundle all bound together. And he commanded them to break the bundle, which none of them could do." As Longo recounts the story, "Artaxerxes" unravels the moral, explaining that the bundle can never be broken if the shafts are tightly bound, but if pulled out one by one, shattering them will be easy. In Longo's retelling, the king's sons prove this to themselves, and their father concludes: "Now you see that if you are one in valor, spirit, and strength, no one will be able to conquer you or break your power. If you are divided, however, your enemies can easily overwhelm you, just like these spear shafts, as you have seen." Thus an old physician taught his sons a lesson about fraternal *unanimitas.*[12]

This was an excellent example to illustrate his point, but the original story did not involve Artaxerxes. Rather, the wise king thus described by Plutarch had been Scilurus, king of the Scythians, whom Plutarch praises in his ironically wordy treatise against loquaciousness, *De garrulitate.*[13] Plutarch's story of Scilurus's bundle of spear shafts appears as he shifts from negative examples—anecdotes about the misfortunes of the garrulous—to positive examples of laudably laconic folk who transmit their meaning "by signs, without a word."[14] Had Longo forgotten that the wise king in question was Scilurus, not Artaxerxes? Perhaps he encountered this story in the course of youthful studies and had not reread it in many years. Or perhaps he had conflated the figures, as it would have been easy to do, because Scilurus appears very near to a mention of Artaxerxes elsewhere in the *Moralia.* He might have been led astray by a printer's error. And, although Longo owned Greek books, he may not have been fully literate in that language.

All are possible explanations, but there is something more interesting in this transposition than faulty readings or erroneous translations. Longo needed the great Persian king. One reason might have been impact: Any reader of the Bible, Plutarch's *Lives* and *Moralia,* Herodotus, or Thucydides would have heard the name Artaxerxes.[15] Longo may also have participated, to a degree, in the common humanist practice of giving redactions of Plutarch's *Lives* to cement patronage and friendship ties—always an appropriate text in these contexts, given the positive models for both governors and citizens that he offered.[16] But Longo also identified with this king, attributing to him an essential exhortation to virtue. What we see here is Longo's participation in a humanist tradition of admiration for "alien wisdom" and specifically for the "wise men of the East" that we consider more closely hereafter.

This identification with Artaxerxes persisted through decades. Longo turned to his Persian model as well in his first will of 1552, which he wrote during an illness. At this moment he had three healthy sons, a daughter who had demonstrated a spiritual vocation that pleased him, and a beloved wife deemed capable of administering his estate, as well as several friends and relatives ready to assist her. Yet this testament, too, expresses a profound fear that his sons might ruin everything by quarreling. Once again, he invokes Artaxerxes as he urges the boys "to be of one spirit and one will" and recounts the story of the spear shafts with its moral in the same way that he would do in his final will. Longo must have felt a real connection with his model, then, as he reached for it in two documents separated by twenty-two years.

His earlier will also has more from the Persian king, another inspiring application of his example—and this time it really was Artaxerxes's example. Longo bequeaths to his younger brother, Girardo, a ring, his "annello da bolla" as he terms it, meaning a ring with a seal or stamp. Longo offered this ring as a "sign of love" to be enjoyed "on account of love," but he was aware that it still might seem too small a gift. Accordingly, he urges his brother to "appreciate more my goodwill than the gift itself, recalling that Artaxerxes, the most famous king of Persia, did not disdain to taste the crystalline waters from a translucent fountain, which had been fetched by the calloused hands of a rough peasant, esteeming as he did the affect and not the effect of drinking the water."[17] Once again, the wise Persian king filled the rhetorical need.[18] Plutarch had originally used this anecdote in dedicating a part of the *Moralia* to the emperor Trajan, urging his dedicatee to follow Artaxerxes in viewing magnanimity as the ability not only to give large gifts but to accept small ones graciously.[19] Longo thus chose an apt classical *topos* for reminding his brother of the virtue of magnanimity.

Longo invested in this material, however, embellishing it with new details. Plutarch's description of the laborer's gift is straightforward: "A simple laborer, possessed of nothing else, took up water in his two hands." Dr. Longo amplified the image, adding a physician's attention to corporality. In Longo's retelling, the "simple laborer" becomes a "rough peasant" *(rozzo villano),* and the offering hands are made more visceral for being "calloused" *(cullose).* So, too, our physician had a humanist's passion for rhetorical contrast. Plutarch concluded simply that Artaxerxes appreciated "the ready goodwill" rather than the "degree of service rendered" by the peasant's gift. Longo expands the idea, observing that Artaxerxes tasted in the water its "affect" and not its "effect" *(l'affetto non l'effetto).* The ideas are Plutarch's in both cases, but Longo appropriated them. He not only collected from antiquity; he connected with it and understood his own world through it.

As Arnaldo Momigliano suggested long ago, the ancient Greeks, even while fighting the Persians, understood the civilization of Persia to be a repository of admirable "alien wisdom."[20] As Margaret Meserve has shown, Renaissance intellectuals followed suit in putting forth a roster of ancient Eastern models for emulation.[21] Paradigmatically, Xenophon's *Cyropaedia* (especially as filtered through Cicero) made Cyrus the "consummate philosopher-prince, paragon of royal wisdom, virtue, piety, political savvy."[22] This tradition persisted even in Machiavelli's *Prince.*[23] Artaxerxes served Francesco Longo as a similar exemplar. Ancient conceptions of Persian valor and unity on the battlefield found their way into sixteenth-century Venetian chronicles and histories that praised the contemporary Ottomans for their exemplary display of *unanimitas.* Venetian humanism and civic rhetoric continually emphasized the virtue of working and fighting as if "of one single will" and used their enemies-cum-trading partners in the East as exemplars when the rhetorical occasion warranted.[24] In the microcosm, so did Francesco Longo, who schooled his sons in unanimity by means of "Artaxerxes."

It is one thing to find citations of wise Persians in the publications of celebrated men of letters, who lived by parading their encyclopedic knowledge; it is another thing to find this comparatist spirit in the final testament of a middling-sort physician. And while Longo's illustrious contemporaries pondered the "wise men of the East" in abstract terms, he claimed membership in that foreign tradition. In Longo's first will, Artaxerxes serves as an example for his brother; in his final will, Artaxerxes became a simulacrum for himself. Like the Persian king, Longo had a number of sons, but one estate. The Longo heirs might well destroy their little empire, too, as they fought to dominate it. Perhaps the only real difference in the cases would be scale.

Longo's lessons highlighted the significance of his experiences, making universal the events of a life that had been ordinary. This physician's choice of Plutarch also tethered his wills to humanistic culture. As noted earlier, the works of Plutarch served as common coin in humanist friendship economies. In particular, younger humanists aiming to ingratiate themselves with potential patrons or with more established colleagues often made recipients gifts of their translations of Plutarch as erudite introductions and displays of literary and philosophical depth.[25]

Longo's self-respect, however, found expression even apart from direct classical quotations (or misquotations). Like many of his social and professional peers, Longo signaled his education and his library multiple times in his testament. We consider these aspects of his testamentary humanism in due course. For the moment, let us concentrate on Longo's persistent use of the ethical bequest and his further reflections on Artaxerxes. His expressions in this line exhibit a general philosophical impulse that curiously parallels both contemporary Jewish wills and ancient Greek models.[26]

In moving toward the conclusion of his last testament, he offered his sons more general life advice. He urged Pietro and Cornelio to avoid giving loans of money or anything else to anyone without first considering the likelihood that they and the objects of their intended generosity would "become enemies on account of that loan" or else that the loan will never be repaid. "This sort of thing," Longo admits, "has happened to me more than once." Still, he continues, "so as not to lack charity, lend up to five ducats to a person who seems even dearer to you than a friend or a relative—if indeed it is possible that such a person could ever find themselves in need in the first place. But immediately forget about that loan, as if it were something you had never done."[27]

Having dispensed with financial ethics, Longo makes one last bequest to his sons. In the testamentary space reserved for charitable bequests, Longo bequeathed a crash course in Christian Stoicism. "Finally, I urge you to turn to God Omnipotent, Our Lord Jesus Christ," he concludes, "frankly asking him to take your side in all of your endeavors, great and small. Be kind to all, but flatterers to none and familiar with few. Be very slow to anger, but swift to forgiveness and piety. In adversity, be patient; in prosperity, be continent. And in all of your actions be prudent, humble, and crafty."[28] This concatenation of *sententiae,* which sounds so much like the garrulous court adviser Polonius in Shakespeare's *Hamlet,* is both characteristic of Longo's historical moment and not. In an age in which merchant account books routinely begin "in the name of God and profit" and fifty years on from Machiavelli's *The Prince,* counseling piety and craftiness in the same breath was not necessarily a contradiction. Nor was there anything odd about enlisting the Almighty as "second" in one's quotidian duels. It is more unusual, however, to find a list of Stoic precepts wedged into the concluding lines of a will, where testators were expected to specify gifts to convents, monasteries, hospitals, the poor, or other charitable causes. For a man of learning, however, wisdom freely offered might be a form of charity; it certainly served as proof of philosophy. Longo's strong self-conception as a philosopher links him to one ancient tradition compellingly reinterpreted for us in recent years by Pierre Hadot. Focused on Marcus Aurelius, Hadot recovers the elements that formed the model of the Stoic philosopher that inspired many aspirants in succeeding centuries, including Longo: the use of personal experiences as spurs to contemplate universal principles; focusing an enlivening philosophical rumination by close attention to political models; the technique of repeating aphorisms from the Stoic canon; appreciation of the "psychological power of the well-turned phrase"; and a conception of ethical memoranda as a form of inheritance.[29]

If Longo deserved credit for mimicking (consciously or not) the philosopher-emperor, he deserved even more for devoting greater attention than Marcus did to governing his children. Longo hoped that his heirs would protect, perpetuate, and bring honor to the family. And he had a particular vision for how they might proceed. As we have learned, his sons must remain united and, to the extent possible, adopt a Stoic attitude toward the vicissitudes of fortune. He urged piety as well, of course, but only in conjunction with his other precepts. Longo's philosophy also encompassed a conception of teleological ethics and an insistence on the virtues of self-reliance and industry much akin to that of Massa and other practitioners of testamentary humanism.

These forms of philosophical bequest inform his instructions in his final will but receive explicit articulation in his first will (1552). In this case, Longo gave his sons a targeted lesson in teleological ethics. Alluding to Machiavelli, he urged all three (this will predated Giulio's affliction) to "keep before [their] eyes the ultimate end of [their] endeavors, because (as a wise man of the world says), whatever has a good conclusion is good and, conversely, whatever ends badly is bad."[30] And, once again in the place commonly reserved for charitable bequests, he left an exhortation. In this case, Longo taught his sons the value of industry. "I entreat my dearest and most beloved sons," he intoned, "to forget that they have any inheritances coming to them, so that they may exert themselves (one in one profession, another in another) to earn their livings, striving always to live by their own industry and virtue."[31] Thus he had counseled them to avoid the lassitude of comfortable heirs and to cherish independence and hard work. Apparently having a "work ethic" did not, in fact, require a Protestant confessional allegiance. Indeed, as we saw in Chapter 1, the philosophical value of hard work inspired comment from two Venetian priests, besides two other physicians (apart from Longo) and a lawyer.

Longo's robust approach to testamentary humanism, spanning direct classical references and multiple ethical bequests, constructed a monument to his learning and the ways he applied it. While he may have written under a pseudonym or his compositions may have been lost, nothing attributed to him either in manuscript or in print has yet been found. He seems, then, not to have proved his cultural honor through publication, as many of his fellow physicians did. And a career in print would have been possible for him, given his education and connections. His extended networks even included one published physician-humanist, Diomedes Bonardo, the first translator of Galen's complete corpus from Greek into Latin (1490).[32] Between the time of his first will (1552) and that of his final will (1574), Longo had taken on the trusteeship of Bonardo's estate, which had formerly been the responsibility of one of his cousins. In Bonardo, Longo would have had an excellent model for the figure of the physician-humanist and his particular modes of self-presentation. Bonardo's brief Latin preface to the translation of Galen notes that he was a practicing physician from Brescia who had "zealously and scrupulously pored over the books of Galen," further accentuating his humanistic credentials in positioning himself, with reference to Plato, as a selfless servant of knowledge. "As God is my witness," he swears, "I have devoted myself to this project not in the hope of monetary gain, but instead supported only by knowledge and truth, thinking that human beings have no better or more divine possession than the truth."[33] With a physician-humanist of Bonardo's type already within his own networks, Longo had an immediate authorial model. Yet he does not seem to have emulated it in this direct way.

Longo's testament, however, does emulate such an ideal at least in his general emphasis on his cultural honor, rather than his professional credentials. He wanted this statement to reflect the passions and pursuits of a philosophical mind not an occupational success story. Many physicians commented in their wills on their status in the medical field. Voicing common requests, Michele di Muti specified that the College should be at full complement for his funeral, his bier should be decorated with the books "commonly placed on us doctors when we are buried," probably indicating his editions of Hippocrates and Galen, and a fellow physician should give the funerary oration instead of a priest.[34] By contrast, Longo forgot to specify his occupation when signing his final will; he inserted the term "physi[c]o" later.[35]

Longo also emphasized his linguistic skills and his doctorates. While his occupational title briefly slipped his mind, he did not neglect to provide a superfluous explanation (as Massa and Superchio did) for why he wrote his will in Italian instead of Latin or to list his full academic title. In both of his wills, he specifies that he was a "Doctor of Arts and Medicine." As Nancy Siraisi reminds us, *Doctor* always meant *university graduate* and was the highest form of address for men in the medical field, who might otherwise be called *medici* (a medical or surgical practitioner) or *physici,* a label similar to our term *general practitioner,* indicating the individual's rank above that of surgeons—specialists at the time held a place well below generalists.[36] We may be sure that Longo's use of his full academic title was a deliberate choice, because not all of his colleagues did so. Maffeo dei Maffei terms himself neither physician nor doctor. Nicolò Massa calls himself simply a "phisico." Even Superchio chose "phisico" in his will proper, but in his codicil he used the phrase that Longo favored. Several other physicians used a shorthand version, "dottor phisico."[37] A good number of physicians, however, shared with Longo the desire to highlight their university degrees. Ottavian Monaldi and Andrea Baranzon also favored the title "Doctor of Arts and Medicine."[38] Women related to physicians also tended to give their relatives' academic titles. In 1534, Fiornovella Balsi, a widow, named the physician Antonio Marin (the husband of her niece) as her principal executor, and in so doing highlighted his doctorates in the liberal arts and in medicine.[39] In 1575, Franceschina, daughter of Nicolò Massa's nephew Apollonio, who was also a physician and twice prior of the College (1549 and 1550), termed her father "The Most Excellent Doctor of Arts and Medicine."[40] Women's social place depended largely on the professions of their fathers, husbands, and even extended male kin and friends, as Fiornovella Balsi's will suggests. That women underscored the university credentials of their male relatives reinforces the power of educational attainments in calculations of a family's honor.

While invoking Persian kings, marginalizing his profession, and emphasizing his doctorates, Longo underscored the breadth of his learning by giving prominent place to consideration of his library. The collection of books he had formed received comment in the last section of bequests before the conclusion. In emphasizing his bibliographic legacy, Longo looks like the many others seeking and finding cultural legitimacy in Renaissance Venice. Longo's statement that his books should never be sold, unlike other valuables he was willing to see parceled out if need arose, highlights the importance he attached to his bibliographic legacy. "My books," Longo insisted, "I will that they not be sold, but to Pietro my son I leave all those in Latin and Greek, and those in Italian I leave to Nonio Cornelio, with this condition: Neither of them may sell or give them away, but instead keep them for their own use and the use of their heirs and descendants." Longo also urged his sons make a careful inventory of the library, then reiterated that the collection must not be in any way alienated until such time as the family line came to an end. In that case, the last descendant might give his book collection "to a monastery that has a library for the friars and others, or indeed to the friars who may be caring for my aforementioned son Giulio."[41]

Longo described his library in terms similar to those Nicolò Massa had used in bequeathing his own collection. Concerned with its preservation, and trusting in his heirs to make an inventory, Longo did not note any particular volumes but did explain that he owned books in Italian, Latin, and Greek. As we know Massa's collection to have covered the same linguistic territories and encompassed more than 100 books, and as physicians' median collection was 140 volumes, Longo's library probably had similar proportions. We also have a household inventory for Longo's eldest son, Pietro, that mentions a full inventory of books, which would likely have included those in Latin and Greek Pietro had received from his father.[42] Unfortunately, the inventory of Pietro Longo's library has not survived, but the fact that Pietro had one made suggests the conservation and no doubt augmentation of a family collection with substantial proportions and value. At all events, Longo's concern for his library evinces that he invested his sense of cultural worth in the volumes he owned in ways akin to other humanistic testators whom we have encountered.

Longo shared with other practitioners of testamentary humanism the desire to leave a record of his cultural no less than material possessions. He offered beneficiaries Artaxerxes (even more than Christ) as a model for magnanimity and unity, and he troubled to incorporate mention of his skill in languages, university degrees, and his library. More idiosyncratically, Longo aimed to show that he lived and died as a moral philosopher and not just a medical doctor. We consider his proofs of conduct further hereafter. But even as distinctive as his rhetoric can be, and as detached as he seems from more usual considerations of "converting" cultural capital into literal advancement, practical realities no doubt influenced, to a degree, Longo's philosophical self-fashioning.

LIVING EDUCATIONAL SOCIAL MOBILITY

I have been arguing that Longo offers a more lyrical approach to his final will and that his claims to cultural legitimacy followed an ethical less than an instrumental program, at least compared with Massa or Superchio. Humanistic studies gave him models that helped him cope with the blows of fortune and that he bequeathed to his beneficiaries and heirs hoping that they would be similarly edified and comport themselves honorably. We have not seen Longo hector his sons about career success, even as he does share with colleagues an insistence on certain virtues, above all independent accumulation of merit. But no human being, however philosophically inclined, exists in a vacuum. Part of the conception of merit obtaining in Longo's family involved education and the opportunities it opened for upward mobility. Longo had experienced that trajectory, even if he did not press his sons to go further, and that experience informed his precepts as much as Plutarch did. Coming from an artisan family, but inhabiting after his university studies a professional zone of metaphorical "nobility," Longo confronted in literal ways the negative assumptions about social climbing. He thus had even more reason to situate himself within the world of abstract merits and be unconcerned with building financial capital beyond that necessary to support his family.

Francesco Longo's father, Pietro, had earned a good reputation as an apothecary and proprietor of a pharmacy called the Testa d'Oro (The Golden Head) in Venice. While Pietro died before Francesco matriculated at the University of Padua, he must have devoted considerable effort and expense to his sons' educations. Both Francesco and his brother Girardo had received sufficient training in Latin to go on to university at the usual ages. Pietro Longo, then, had evidently hoped to position his sons at a higher socioprofessional level than he could occupy.

According to the friends and colleagues who testified on behalf of Francesco Longo's matriculation into the Sacred College of Philosophers and Physicians at the University of Padua in 1530, Pietro Longo had owned a pharmacy in the Campo San Bartolomeo in Venice's Rialto district, the focal point for buying and selling in the city.[43] As a mercantile hub, the Rialto had both the promise and the taint of commerce. Here the city was enriched, but here, too, money changed hands, foreigners mixed freely with citizens, and cultural boundaries blurred. Selling products was compromising enough in terms of social status, but making products of any sort meant classification as a manual laborer and thus exclusion from privileges, including membership in university colleges. Pietro Longo's friends and his son's supporters therefore attempted to classify the elder Longo as a merchant and not an artisan. One witness, a merchant named Acharius Stat, conceded that Pietro Longo began his career as a sort of worker *(tanquam factor)* at one apothecary shop in Venice at the Sign of the Golden Apples but later became something like the owner *(tanquam patronus)* of another at the Sign of the Golden Head.[44] Pelegrino, a Paduan pharmacist, gave Pietro Longo a more advanced entry-level position as the manager *(gubernator)* of the "Golden Apples," though he also emphasized that Longo later set up his own shop at the "Golden Head."[45] A third witness, Pietro, a pharmacist who worked in the same Paduan *bottega* as Pelegrino did, never mentioned the Golden Apples; he simply pointed out that Pietro Longo was the pharmacist at the Golden Head.[46] In their different ways, all the witnesses indicated that Pietro Longo was not a laborer, at least by the end of his career, but a shop owner. The pharmacists Pelegrino and Pietro added for good measure that Pietro Longo was an "man of the right sort" *(uomo da bene),* meaning in this case certainly an honest merchant, but as we have seen in the case of humanistic testators the same term might be connected with cultural attainments. Along these lines, the two pharmacists noted that their old colleague had even done "remarkable things" *(fecce gran facende),* a phrase that in one of its Latin permutations (*magna faciens,* "doing great things") used by humanists connoted magnanimous and charitable service to the public, putting money, skills, and knowledge in the service of the common good.[47] At the very least, Pelegrino and Pietro represented Pietro Longo's activities as well beyond the menial aspects of pharmaceutical work.[48]

The apothecary Pietro Longo had made enough of a mark within his own milieu that his sons had at least a reasonable chance of moving beyond it if they wished. But there were difficulties to be confronted. Pietro Longo did not have university credentials. He was certainly literate, and his education might even have included Latin—possibly even extending to humanistic studies. Among the humanists Lauro Martines found working in Renaissance Florence, there were not many artisans (even higher artisans), but included in those ranks he did locate one notable pharmacist, Matteo Palmieri.[49] At a minimum, a pharmacist would have to read the common herbals, manage his accounts, and write receipts. But the dividing line between the competent and the university educated was carefully policed in the Renaissance. Pietro Longo's reputation as a pharmacist and the money he earned in his trade gave his sons a good, but not optimal, point of origin.

Pietro Longo's second son, Girardo, took his father's place in the family pharmacy, but none of the testimonials mention that. Alessandro Rugerio, a secretary in the Venetian chancery, explained that Girardo Longo had also served as a secretary for the Venetian government.[50] Other documents tell a different story. In his final will, Francesco Longo forgave several debts owed to the family pharmacy that were recorded in his own account books "and those of my brother, up to the time of my brother's death."[51] In 1556, Girardo Longo witnessed the will of a tailor, for whom he would also serve as executor, specifying his occupation at that time as "spitier alla Testa d'Oro" (pharmacist at the Golden Head).[52] Had Girardo Longo simply been the owner of the shop, he probably would not have called himself a pharmacist. And if he wished to specify an occupation for clarity's sake, why did he not call himself a secretary? Perhaps Girardo continued to be involved in both endeavors, but identified himself with the family pharmacy because his name remained associated with the *bottega* and not the chancery. His secretarial post may even have been short term.

I relate these different accounts of Pietro Longo's activities and the apparent contradiction in Girardo's career not to set up a discovery of some document that reveals what Francesco Longo's relatives did with their days. I have found no such evidence. Rather, what we need to appreciate is that these witnesses, testifying in favor of Francesco Longo's acceptance into the medical college at Padua, engaged in selective reporting. Pietro and Girardo Longo might have played any number of roles in the family *bottega* as owners, accountants, pharmaceutical authorities, or even grinders of spices. Yet witnesses emphasized the end of Pietro Longo's career and spoke of Girardo Longo only as a secretary, a man with a "civil" profession. Pharmacists, like notaries, ranked at the highest level of artisans. But the pharmaceutical trade suggested manual activity and thus might have compromised Francesco Longo's candidacy. These testimonials, then, reinforce the constraints of social hierarchy in Renaissance Venice while at the same time indicating that there were methods for crossing from one category to the next.

Merit, real and represented, enabled mobility.[53] Witnesses' emphasis on Pietro Longo's ownership of his shop pushed aside the image of an artisan wielding a mortar and pestle, which he would unavoidably have done at some point, even if only during his apprenticeship. Presenting Pietro Longo instead as a man with real achievements to his credit, witnesses concurred that he was an honest proprietor who also did "great things," an impressive (and usefully vague) compliment. The possibility that Girardo Longo ever worked with his hands never became an issue, thanks to Rugerio's testimony that Longo merited a secretarial post.

Francesco Longo's university degrees, no less than his brother's government work, multiplied the family's portfolio of cultural assets by orders of magnitude. By the sixteenth century, humanists had destabilized conceptions of "nobility," claiming that this quality hinged less on blood than on "virtue," meaning both Christian morality and classical accomplishments.[54] Paradigmatically, we have Poggio Bracciolini's *De vera nobilitate*.[55] The ideal of the "Renaissance man," initially promulgated in elegant Latin treatises such as Bracciolini's, became ubiquitous in Cinquecento literature, finding its most popular expression in Baldassare Castiglione's best seller, *The Courtier*. While no enemy of the titles and inherited wealth on display in the Mantuan court he served, Castiglione emphasized that blood could only be one part of nobility, the fullest embodiment of which required familiarity with ancient and modern languages and literatures, artistic and musical genres, military skills, and the art of conversation. Castiglione also considered possession of these refinements an asset for advancement at court.

Men and women living in the more flexible social world of urban centers could be even more certain that intellectual and cultural credentials repaid their acquisition. University degrees entailed social privileges. Doctors of arts, law, and medicine received the honorific title "Eccellente" ("Your Excellency" or "The Eminent"). By contrast, even the most renowned pharmacist, notary, jurist, or merchant would only be termed "Spettabile" ("The Noteworthy"). The difference may seem subtle, but its significance was crucial in a social world as theoretically precise in its categories as Renaissance Italy. Holders of university degrees also enjoyed sumptuary and connubial concessions. Lawyers and physicians were permitted to wear velvet and long sleeves, sartorial status markers that were otherwise reserved for the nobility. Lawyers and physicians could also marry patrician women. Titles followed the patriline, so the sons of such unions would not be patricians. Daughters of these unions stood a good chance of making patrician matches, however, and their children would be noble. While a lawyer or a physician could not sit in the Great Council, then, or see their surname inscribed into the famous *Libro d'Oro* (the roll call of patrician families), close association with the nobility and even patrician grandchildren were possibilities. And university graduates might themselves be taken for patricians, given their apparel.

The newly minted Dr. Longo had access, by virtue of his degrees, to different social worlds than his father inhabited. Pietro Longo's friends and colleagues included the merchant Acharius Stat and the Paduan pharmacists Pelegrino and Pietro, whose surnames (if they had any) the university's rectors and scribes did not deem worth recording. By contrast, Pietro Longo's sons counted as associates men in the legal profession, for instance, Secretary Rugerio. Already a man with a civil profession, Rugerio seems to have had mobility in mind for himself as well: He was available to testify, because he was happened to be at the University of Padua in 1530, working for the doctorate in law that would earn him more illustrious posts. Francesco Longo's years at Padua naturally extended his and his family's social networks even further.

Longo's career, given his natal family, still necessitated powerful support. Among his most important mentors was Francesco Bonafede, an established member of the medical faculty and the first physician-scholar to lecture on pharmacology. Bonafede would also prove useful to the university in his petitions to the Venetian Senate to approve the construction of a formal botanical garden, which was established in 1545–1546 and remains one of the university's claims to fame.[56] Bonafede had taken his medical degree not from Padua but from the College of Physicians in Venice in 1506 and had served in 1515 as prior of the College. Fifteen years later, he was well established in the more prestigious faculty of medicine at Padua and serving as a *promotor* (committee member) and examiner for doctoral candidates. Longo's own *promotor* for his arts degree in 1530 and an examiner for his medical degree in 1535, Bonafede played a crucial role in furthering Longo's career. After his doctorates, Francesco Longo was immediately admitted to the College of Venice "senza ballotazione" (without the usual formal vote) in 1531.[57] Longo would serve twice as the College's treasurer (1534 and 1543) and twice as its prior (1535 and 1559).[58] Like any other young physician, Longo needed connections; however, as one whose background linked him to the world of apothecaries, whom physicians considered it their special mandate to regulate, control, and police, he needed them all the more. Longo's swift progress through *cursus honorum* of an institution that privileged seniority attests to the importance of his connection to Bonafede.[59]

Further suggestion for the difficulties attendant to intellectual social mobility and the need for supporters among the enfranchised derives from the very sources we have been considering that attest to Longo's time at Padua. These records form part of an unusual *processo* (inquiry) concerning his social background that took place during his matriculation into the college of physicians for doctoral work. The inquiry focused on two sensitive topics: his citizenship and his legitimacy. It is possible that someone had questioned the suitability of a pharmacist's son for membership in this rarified world. Assaults on intellectuals often took the same form as those on anybody else, targeted attacks on family honor.[60] Fortunately, the citizenship question had an easy resolution: Secretary Rugerio was Venetian and argued, rightly, that Girardo Longo could not have served as a secretary in the *Signoria* without verification that his father had been a Venetian citizen.[61] But the biological legitimacy question left everyone stumped. The parish priest of San Giacomo dell'Orio, in a note dated the same day as the questioning, averred that Pietro Longo was born in his parish and held by the community to be a Venetian citizen. Yet he conceded that there were no written records attesting the legitimacy of Longo's sons.[62] He would not have been alone in these days before the Council of Trent clarified marriage and baptismal and related protocols. Acharius Stat, the German merchant, was more helpful in attesting to the sexual propriety of the Longo patriarch. A self-described friend of Pietro Longo "for something like thirty-six years," Stat averred that his friend was held in the mercantile community as a *uomo da bene,* which in this case probably also indicated honesty in business dealings. Stat also emphasized that at least one—and possibly both—of Pietro Longo's sons had been baptized. Stat had stood as godfather, he explains, "either for Francesco or for his brother—or maybe both of them—I can't remember exactly."[63] This evidence was far from watertight, but it was evidently sufficient for a noncriminal investigation.

The rectors had room to deny Francesco Longo full membership in the sodality of medical students, had they wished to do so. They did not wish to do so and, indeed, may have looked on the proceedings as a formality. Yet the tensions here reinforce the notion that identity and status in the early-modern world were fragile and contingent. The testimonials also give us some hint of the difficulties that people faced as they changed social categories. Mobility was possible, but it would require discursive finesse and reliable social networks.

In short, Francesco Longo needed help in his university and professional career. To shift places from the higher artisanal or, at best, mercantile world of a pharmacist to the civil ranks required root-level support. It also required effort, as the wills of Longo, Nicolò Massa, and other humanistic testators have emphasized. And the slights and struggles attendant to that mobility left a desire and a need to continue proving cultural legitimacy. If his father had been deemed a *uomo da bene* primarily in the sense of being an honest merchant, in positioning himself Longo needed to emphasize his intellectual and not merely mercantile honor. But what about his children?

LONGO'S CHILDREN: CRUCIBLES FOR MORAL PHILOSOPHY

Francesco Longo represented his children as the greatest tests of his Christian Stoicism and, by that same token, ultimately the means of proving that he lived his ethical ideals. As Christopher Celenza has shown, it was exemplary living, informed by classical precepts, that defined the project of philosophy in the Italian Renaissance.[64] Longo did not have anything like Marsilio Ficino's philological mastery, but he shared his general objective. As we listen to him attempting to secure the well-being of his heirs,

Longo emerges more fully human, as someone fighting, and not always succeeding, to maintain the hope that he could by force of will and rhetoric provide for the future.

Among the many troubles assailing his eudemonia was the likelihood that Pietro and Nonio Cornelio would fight, in the process rending the little estate by which he himself might be remembered: "I hereby declare that my desire is to put in order these possessions, however small they may be, so that after my death my descendants and heirs will have no reason to litigate against each other, but instead will live harmoniously. And this I exhort and pray above all else: that they will keep among themselves the peace that Our Lord Jesus Christ left to his disciples and to all of us; and that they will content themselves with what I have ordained; and that they will conduct themselves like loving brothers and my dearest sons."[65] Longo's anti-litigation clause is standard fare in Venetian wills of the era, but his expansive comments on this theme, his invocation of Christ's peace, and the fulsome explication suggest a pronounced anxiety on the point. He had reasonable cause for such a fear, as he would be asking his two capable sons to care for an incapacitated brother, as well as a sister at a convent.

What ailed Giulio Longo? Sometime between 1552 and 1574, Giulio began to exhibit behaviors that in his father's estimation necessitated external control. In 1552, Longo made Giulio a coheir and executor of his will alongside his other sons. In 1574, Giulio had become a charity case for Pietro and Nonio Cornelio (or else a monastery) to manage, and he was removed from any role in administering Longo's estate. In 1552, Giulio would have been in adolescence, so if his father had decided to maintain the integrity of the properties by disinheriting a superfluous son, he could have done so at this time.[66] Longo's financial situation in 1574 had not become appreciably more perilous than it had been in 1552, which might have prompted this drastic approach to estate planning. Even as late as 1566, apparently Giulio's difficulties had not manifested. In that year, his mother bequeathed to him an equal share of her dotal funds without further comment.[67] Apparently something happened to Giulio Longo between 1566 and 1574 that affected him mentally, emotionally, physically, or some combination thereof. It is not difficult to imagine such a calamity. Plague, syphilis, to say nothing of the usual array of accidents, left their mark on any number of Giulio's contemporaries. We also know that his elder brother, Pietro, went blind toward the end of his life, so it is not impossible that a congenital disorder might have struck Giulio earlier.[68]

I incline toward an explanation less physical than psychological, as Longo becomes uncharacteristically vague when discussing Giulio's troubles. He begins by saying that only Pietro and Nonio Cornelio should take care of his funeral arrangements, because "Giulio is, by nature, unsuited to such tasks." Thereafter, Longo specifies that his real estate must remain a solid unit under the joint administration of Pietro and Cornelio. "I do not want Giulio to have any part in the decision making," he explains, "because he is not fit for this sort of thing, as is obvious."[69] Thus far, we get the impression that Giulio simply had no head for business. Further on in the testament, however, Longo stipulates that Pietro and Cornelio must watch over their brother on pain of disinheritance. This serves as a point of departure for an extended disquisition on Giulio's situation:

> You must take care of your brother, Giulio, taking on his expenses, "putting him in clothes and shoes" as the saying goes, and looking after him jointly in a brotherly way—in your home, if you choose to live together, or, if not, in the household of whichever of you he wishes to live with, caring for him as brothers must do. I make this a condition, because Giulio is completely incompetent; he cannot even control himself, as is clear to many people. Let him live out his days together with you and with whatever dignity he can. This I command, demand, and entreat you to do, in the bowels of Christ, bearing in mind that if God had allowed it to happen, you and indeed all of us might have found ourselves to be far worse than that which he is—being as all of us are created by nature—as one sees clearly in many other cases.[70]

Longo does not quite give a diagnosis, but something close to it. He refers to his son as a "case" like many others. He allows that Giulio's afflictions were perceptible, being "obvious" or "noted" by many people, and (in his haunting clause "that which he is") he suggests that these afflictions had altered Giulio's very being. Most important, Longo points to natural accident as the real source of the problem ("all of us are created by nature"), suggesting that humans, as physical creatures, are to a certain degree at the mercy of external forces beyond their control. What had happened to Giulio, he reasons, could have happened to anyone. Indeed, Longo shows himself to be a man of his profession in emphasizing the role of nature more than divine will. He does not say that the Almighty willed or ordained Giulio's difficulty; at most the Supreme Being "might have let it happen."

Longo's remarks exhibit his general philosophical tendency toward making universal meaning out of particular cases, but here he does so in a vein that connects him to discourses on ailments current in his profession. The published works of sixteenth-century physicians perform the same theoretical contortions in their explanations of the causes of disease and the role of the physician in addressing them. Medical authors concede to divine will while emphasizing the power of nature and representing the physician as a mediator capable (God willing) of manipulating the natural world—the patient's body and the herbs and unguents to be administered on it—in remedying illness and injury. Longo's illustrious colleague Trincavella had emphasized the physician's limited agency in noting that nature ultimately governs the bodily humors; in manipulating them, the physician is either nothing with respect to nature or else simply her collaborator *(medicus vero, aut nihil aut parum).* Trincavella cautioned his readers that the physician does nothing without the help of nature's power in general and the particular manifestation of that power in the patient's "innate heat" *(calor nativus),* or life force. Still, the physician can, through medicaments, work to reestablish humoral equilibrium and "in so doing can assist nature as (so to speak) her helper and attendant."[71] In his attempts to parse the roles played by nature, accident, and God's will in the course of his son's afflictions, Longo joined his colleagues.

Naturally, the problem of physicians' limited agency became all the more anguishing as the "case" here was Longo's own son. Adding a painful measure of irony to the situation, moreover, the physician's chief responsibilities included assisting their patients with maintaining or returning to a philosophical equilibrium that might, together with diet, exercise, and other tangible helps, catalyze a return to humoral balance. In speaking of Giulio and his condition, then, Longo confronted his uncertainty as to causes. He thought perhaps God had "let it happen," or perhaps nature was more to blame. The possibility of witchcraft had evidently also occurred to this worried father, as he remarks that Giulio must never be left to handle any affairs by himself as he might easily fall prey to "some evildoing [*maleficio*], either of his own or of others."[72] While the context of the sentence suggests the best rendering of this term would be *evildoing* or *malfeasance,* it could certainly also mean an evil spell. Given recent work on conceptions of witchcraft in early-modern Europe, we should not be surprised that Longo gestures toward this occult explanation.[73] But thanks to the work of Jonathan Seitz, neither should we be surprised to see a physician treading so delicately around the topic. As Seitz has shown, physicians called to testify in court whether an unfortunate occurrence, such as a death or miscarriage, had natural or supernatural causes often shifted the burden of discernment onto others, insisting (in good academic manner) that the subject was not really their field and that clerics instead should be asked to judge.[74]

But while Longo's reticence in deciding what ailed Giulio echoed his colleagues' similar reluctance, he could not leave the matter there. Something had to be done with his middle son, and that something needed to accord with his personal ethics but also still have some hope of implementation by his other two sons. As ever, Longo tells us of his deliberations. Giulio had often expressed the desire to enter a monastery, he notes, and he took that eventuality into consideration. While his first choice remained that Giulio should live with one or both of his brothers, he does not forbid his son to take vows. But he worried that Giulio might not be capable of understanding such a decision or communicating it clearly to his brothers. "If ever Giulio truly wishes to go, as he has often said, into a monastery," Longo counsels Pietro and Nonio Cornelio, "in that case—his wishes being clearly understood and the issue rigorously considered both by him and by you two—I advise you to go ahead and monachate him, giving to the brethren where you have placed him the alms that seem best to you. Take care, however . . . that your donation be of a sort to give the brothers good reason to keep him and be good company for him, and make him happy to stay there."[75] He also stipulates that if Giulio becomes a monk, he is to receive eight ducats per year to spend as he likes. Longo's ongoing attempts to explain his thought processes, his deliberations, show us the strain that Giulio's malady put on his father, in particular his efforts to be punctilious in avoiding coercive paternal action.

If Longo's own philosophical equanimity had been tested, he knew that his other sons would have their possibly far more fragile fraternal solidarity burdened near or past the breaking point in caring for Giulio. Hence the need to provide them with the best lesson he could devise: Artaxerxes and the spear shafts, the same story that he had offered his sons in his first will, terming it at that time "a bequest of memorandum and precept."[76] That precept had become all the more crucial in the intervening years, as serious problems arose.

Before we take our leave of Giulio Longo, who (alas) has left no documentary trail of his own, it is worth pausing to consider what his appearances in his father's will tells us about early-modern attitudes toward illness, affliction, even madness. Following Michel Foucault, historians long posited that early-modern European families off-loaded "damaged" relatives as quickly as possible onto charitable institutions, whether hospitals or monasteries.[77] By contrast, Longo's efforts to protect Giulio, to ensure not only his son's basic comfort but also his dignity and even happiness (at least the "good company" of his fellow monks, in the event that he entered a monastery) support new work in the history of medicine and madness that emphasizes a diversity of coping strategies and viewpoints, an argument most recently advanced by Elizabeth Mellyn.[78] Longo modeled compassion and demanded the same from his sons. That Longo felt compelled to put his instructions regarding Giulio into the binding language of Christ's viscera, and furthermore adduced the authority of an ancient Persian king, suggests that he knew his attitude might seem strange or even objectionable; he needed to bolster it. While Longo's singular case, then, cannot in itself give the lie to the old notion that madness and illness were "criminalized" in the early-modern world, he does reinforce the notion that alternative viewpoints were available and put into practice.

Nor did this philosopher-physician exhaust his stores of paternal goodwill on the unfortunate Giulio. Another of Longo's aims in his final will was to ensure the well-being of his daughter, Virginia, who had entered the convent of Corpus Domini more than a decade previously (around 1562). His actions regarding his monachated daughter teach us much the same lessons as those regarding the afflicted Giulio. Scholars traditionally claimed that nuns, even more than married women, became effectively dead to their natal families.[79] Recent research has demolished this view, pointing to many cases of care in the choice of convents and, beyond monachation, continued contact between nuns and their birth kin.[80] The case of Suor Virginia fits this newer conception of relations between nuns and their families.

Francesco Longo placed his daughter at what we might safely consider one of Venice's more prestigious convents. Assessing Corpus Domini's precise rank among the dozens of Venetian convents is tricky. Some scholars situate it as an effectively patrician convent, noting that the family names of its nuns "read like a roll call of Venice's ruling elite, resonant with wealth and glory . . . [Nuns bore the] patrician surnames of doges, admirals, and senators [that] would have been obvious to any Venetian."[81] Others have remarked that Corpus Domini seems, at least by the sixteenth century, to exhibit more social heterogeneity than other Venetian convents, one indication of its diversity being a 1560 ruling by Venice's ecclesiastical authority, Patriarch Giovanni Trevisan, that "girls who were either illegitimate or of artisan stock could not be accepted as choir nuns."[82] Trevisan's ruling suggests that Corpus Domini may have made some women from lower social ranks full members of the chapter. Indeed, Longo's daughter was one of them, technically speaking, although his professional status, perhaps together with his promises of future medical services, may have constituted sufficient grounds for classifying Suor Virginia as "citizen" rank.

Corpus Domini held a place in the convent hierarchy well under that of Santa Maria degli Vergini, whose abbess ceremonially wed the doge each year and whose nuns, exclusively patrician women, regularly wrote and delivered Latin orations.[83] Still, Corpus Domini was recognized as a venerable "ancient" convent (it had been consecrated in 1394) and boasted a sorority of women largely from patrician and citizen families that had considerable clout. Suor Virginia Longo, lacking patrician blood, could not serve as abbess, an elected position held on a rotating basis by the nuns who derived from the city's first families. But she enjoyed a place among the choir nuns who constituted the governing body of the convent. Suor Virginia appears regularly with her peers, convened to witness the most important legal and financial transactions in the convent's daily life. The nuns were assembled, for instance, when a wealthy novice took the veil and the convent received the money or property pledged by her family as her "spiritual dowry." Thanks to this practice, we find Suor Virginia's presence recorded by the notaries alongside approximately forty other nuns from 1562 to her death in 1607.[84]

Longo chose a convent that had considerable cultural cachet and a history related to his own line of work. Corpus Domini had its own internal pharmacy and a tradition of women physicians. At least according to the surviving account books, which commence in the late seventeenth century, Corpus Domini salaried an external physician but also employed one nun as a resident pharmacist, terming her "Mother Apothecary."[85] Early-modern convents necessarily capitalized on the skills that entering nuns brought with them from home. Galileo's daughter Suor Maria Celeste, a nun at the convent of San Matteo in Florence, had received considerable scientific education from her father and became the convent's apothecary.[86] It seems likely that Suor Virginia, growing up in a family of pharmacists-cum-physicians, would similarly have learned a good deal about medicine and may have served as "Mother Apothecary" during her lifetime. As to Corpus Domini's known women healers, we learn from Suor Bartolommea Riccoboni's chronicle that Suor Lucia Tiepolo's earnings from her medical work funded the initial construction of the convent: "She happened to have some money that she had earned by practicing medicine (she treated great crowds of sick people), and with these funds she paid for the land and the lumber and began to have the church constructed out of wood."[87]

It also seems that, like his colleague Superchio, Longo managed to parley his reputation as a man of medicine and learning into situating Virginia well—perhaps also providing his daughter with an education or set of skills that would serve as additional leverage. If Longo paid to Corpus Domini only the three hundred ducats that he had set aside, Suor Virginia's placement as a choir nun would have necessitated additional compensation, for instance, the promise of free medicines or medical consultations from him, or her own potential to make useful contributions to the community. By the early seventeenth century, the spiritual dowry required for choir nuns was fixed at eight hundred to one thousand ducats. By contrast, three hundred ducats constituted the dowry of a *conversa,* a lay nun who worked in the convent as a servant.[88] Clearly, other assets or promises had been involved in Suor Virginia's monachation at Corpus Domini.

Given that for a man in Longo's modest circumstances it was a mark of cultural legitimacy in its own way to have his daughter take her vows at one of the city's better convents, we might suspect that Suor Virginia had fallen victim to family strategy. To be sure, Longo avoided paying the astronomical sums that marrying her to a patrician would have entailed. Patrician dowries often crested the twenty-thousand-ducat mark during this sixteenth century, and a few sixty-thousand-ducat dowries were reported.[89] Seeking a patrician match for a daughter outside its ranks might have required even more. As Jutta Sperling has demonstrated, dowry inflation was so rampant by the turn of the seventeenth century that patrician families began to commit demographic suicide by monachating most or all of their daughters.[90] More humble families also felt the effects of dowry inflation. Consider the four-thousand-ducat dowry that the pharmacist Orfeo Copacio assembled for his daughter, also named Virginia, in the late sixteenth century.[91] A few decades earlier, one thousand or fifteen hundred ducats would easily have secured an advantageous match for her. The spiritual dowry Longo set aside for his daughter was a relative bargain.

Yet this does not seem to be a case of forced monachation, a common problem in the day. In his 1552 will, Dr. Longo describes his daughter's vocation at some length. "Because my daughter Virginia, inspired by God, desires and intends to become a nun and marry Jesus Christ," he explains, "and since I have no intention of contravening her wishes, knowing truly that this is divine inspiration, given her innate goodness, exemplary conduct, and holy manner of life—that is, to dedicate herself wholly to the service of Jesus Christ—I beg my executors, if I have not yet placed her in a convent before I die, to satisfy my little girl's wishes as quickly as possible."[92] We are still in the days before the Council of Trent's rulings on consent in secular marriages and monastic vows (1563), so there was no pressing need for Longo to put words of vocation into his daughter's mouth, as some families did in succeeding decades. Longo seemed, if anything, reluctant to have his daughter leave home. Corpus Domini's records indicate that Virginia Longo did not take her vows there until sometime shortly before or in the year 1562, when her name appears last in the list of chapter nuns present to witness the monachation of a new nun—lists invariably arranged by seniority.[93] Virginia Longo would have remained at home, then, for nearly a decade after her father's 1552 will. And Longo's concern for her welfare persisted until his own death. He left his daughter a small lifetime annuity of five ducats, and he bequeathed an annuity of another ducat to her friend, Suor Theodosia, explaining, "Even though this is so little—indeed, almost nothing—compared to what she deserves for the love she bears toward my daughter, still, I do this to show that I have her in my thoughts, not as recompense for her merits."[94] He also forgave Corpus Domini's old debts to the family pharmacy, he explained, "because of the loving kindness and goodness of those nuns [and] so that my daughter, a nun in that convent, may be treated lovingly, as she has been to this point."[95]

Longo's heirs and executors, Pietro and Nonio Cornelio, would need to effectuate these annuities to their sister and her friend, much as they would be directly responsible for their brother's care. Longo worried about his "superfluous" children and specifically whether his designated heirs would live up to his ethical standards in looking after them. Small wonder, then, that he went to such trouble to put these two sons in a suitably virtuous frame of mind. As we have seen, he urged them to live together in peace and to be "prudent, humble, and crafty" in all their endeavors.[96] He also exhorted them to look always to the final results of their projects.[97] And he offered them the example of Artaxerxes to keep them mindful of the ancient model he had found steadying and inspiring. He did not press them about their studies or specify the occupations they must pursue. His primary concern, leaving questions of social ascent aside, was that they not quarrel and not behave as heirs but instead exert themselves, earning their livelihoods by their own "industry and virtue."[98] In other words, Longo situated family complexities and even tragedies not as "hassles and headaches" in the way that Nicolò Massa did, but instead as crucibles for his own moral philosophy and for that of his sons.

Longo was a man of his era in certain respects, but he did not exhibit many of its common forms of ambition. He did not marry a patrician woman, as his degrees entitled him to do and as some of his peers did. Longo's wife, Marietta, had brought a fifteen-hundred-ducat dowry with her, which was a substantial sum of money but still an artisan-level dowry. Longo apparently valued other things more. Nor did he browbeat his heirs about professional or financial advancement; he lectured them on ethics.[99] In the end, Longo's conception of his posterity had less to do with the usual markers of success and more with a proof that in him and in his family learning and exemplary conduct were indeed as mutually sustaining as humanists claimed.

Marking his belonging in the more particular world of teleological ethics, where results trump intentions in assessment, Longo let us watch him think through and attempt to ensure courses of action that would have positive outcomes. He spoke not of his good intentions, and still less of his submission to divine will. Instead, through force of his own will and rhetoric, he labored to ensure that Giulio "live[d] out his life with as much dignity as possible" and that the nuns of Corpus Domini would continue to treat his daughter lovingly. What Longo was like on a day-to-day basis we cannot know, but in his numerous departures from testamentary formulae he made a convincing case that his studies had helped him forge a link between erudite learning and ethical living that even heartbreak could not rupture.

POSTERITY FOR A PHYSICIAN AND MORAL PHILOSOPHER

Francesco Longo did not represent himself primarily as a member of the medical community, but thanks to his degrees and the early death of his brother, this branch of the family was now associated with that field more than any other. And Longo's kin understood the enhancements he had made, specifically as a physician, to the family's cultural portfolio. Basegio di Lazari, Longo's maternal uncle, made Longo an executor of his testament in 1539. Lazari specified that Francesco Longo was "a doctor of arts and medicine."[100] As a name and relationship would have sufficed to indicate which nephew Lazari meant, it seems that Lazari was proud of Francesco, who was the first member of the patriline to earn a doctorate. Longo's wife, Marietta, while not quite so precise as other physicians' wives, still described her husband as "His Excellency, the physician Francesco Longo."[101]

Longo's line continued, primarily but not exclusively in the world of medicine. Giulio Longo disappears from the records immediately after Longo's final will and the eldest, Pietro, died without issue. But Longo's youngest, Nonio Cornelio, had at least one heir. The trusteeship of the estate of Longo's uncle, Basegio di Lazari, ultimately passed to an Orazio Longo, who appears in the financial records of Corpus Domini to confirm the conclusion of the annual payments on behalf of Suor Virginia in 1609, after the deaths of Virginia herself and her brother Pietro.[102] Although Pietro Longo had no living children at the time of his death and had also spent the last decade of his life unable to practice as a physician owing to blindness, he had formed important ties both within and outside his profession that give his story a less melancholy conclusion. The inventory of Pietro Longo's household goods and papers was performed at the behest of his executors, "Their Excellencies" Antonio Marin and Pietro di Schietti. Schietti must have been a close friend, as he had taken Longo into his own home for care. The assessors note that Schietti had returned a portion of Pietro Longo's cash and clothing to Longo's principal residence from Schietti's own house, where Longo had "passed to the better life."[103] Assessors also noted that the inventory was discussed and ratified at the house of

"His Excellency, Paulo Pincio" (the humanistic priest with the talented illegitimate son whom we met in Chapter 2) with Pincio and another university man, Marco Bastiani, serving as witnesses. Pietro Longo, then, moved in circles of university graduates and had clearly formed more than collegial ties with some of them.

Where Longo's descendants might have gone from there and what other pursuits they may have undertaken we cannot know. The records fall silent. And so the story of the rise of this family from artisans to a civil profession by way of university ends here. The last record of Francesco Longo's existence is a note in the civic necrologies for the year 1576: "His Excellency, messer Francesco di Longo, physician, died of fevers on the 26th of August."[104] As a sign of respect, the notary euphemized the cause of Longo's death as "fevers." By contrast, the tens of thousands Venetians expiring around him were noted either as dead from plague or under suspicion of it. Given what we have seen of Longo's character, it seems unlikely that he would have been much pleased with this deference to his profession. But he would surely have taken satisfaction in learning that his son Pietro remained mindful of his father, and perhaps also of his father's last thoughts. In the inventory of Pietro Longo's possessions and papers made after his death in 1608, assessors noted that atop the bureau in Pietro's own bedroom was "a terracotta portrait of the late Signore Francesco Longo."[105] The diminutive nature of this memorial would likely have struck Longo, who insisted on the vanity and wastefulness of funerary pomp, as more appropriate than the elaborate monument that Maria Massa Grifalcone had commissioned for her father—to say nothing of the self-display in which Longo's colleague Tommaso Rangone indulged, commissioning a large and elaborate bronze statue of himself replete with books, astrolabe, and all the other appurtenances of his profession.[106] One small portrait bust on a bureau, together with his own words on the pages of his testament, sufficed for his memorialization.

Longo's own paper monument expands our conception of the ways in which a sixteenth-century Venetian might understand, seek, and use cultural legitimacy. Some of his contemporaries revealed their literary belonging in vast libraries, or illustrious careers and print publications; however, we can see a similar set of priorities in an ordinary doctor's ethical bequests. Indeed, cultural life emerges in even less promising media. If Nicolò Massa left images of himself as a man of letters in print as well as in reams of family papers, and Longo at least sketched philosophical self-portraits in two ornately rhetorical testaments, their colleague Alberto Rini found room even in his cramped ledgers to record the life of his mind.

CHAPTER 5

CULTURAL LIFE IN THE JOURNALS OF ALBERTO RINI

Inventories and testaments have shown us strong commitments to books, education, and literary ideals across an impressive spectrum of Venetian society. Fighting for personal intellectual honor, the ennoblement of their profession, or even just for their own peace of mind, our physician protagonists have proved especially interesting historical subjects in their varied quests for and experiences of cultural legitimacy. As eloquent as posthumous inventories and final testaments can be, however, by nature they teach us more about individuals' last years and hopes for a reputational afterlife than about their daily lives. What did our physicians' worlds look like at moments when they were not necessarily forced to confront their mortality? Compared with many early-modern Europeans, educated medical doctors had greater access to media in which they might leave traces of their existence, but that relative advantage was ultimately slim. As a rule, the normal, habitual, and everyday simply leave fainter documentary trails than the unusual, dramatic, or final.

This chapter analyzes an exception to that rule, the daily memoranda of the physician Alberto Rini. To contextualize and better appreciate the historical treasures that Rini provides us, however, we should consider a few other sources through which we might learn about early-modern Italian medical doctors, even when we cannot find their inventories, testaments, or other family papers.

If we want to trace the changes in early-modern medical knowledge and practice, we have an abundance of physicians' printed disputations, treatises, and letters, as well as archival material from universities, colleges of physicians, hospitals, civic boards of health, and princely courts where many medical doctors made their careers.[1] As literary critics have illustrated, moreover, drama and poetry also reveal contemporary perceptions of physicians and the different meanings attached to individual diseases as well as to the concept of healing.[2] Getting close to the quotidian, as ever, represents a greater but not an insurmountable challenge. Gianna Pomata has delved into legal records, especially contracts, and found that the relationship between physician and patient was negotiated in all senses of the term: Physicians did not proscribe from on high, as print material often repressed them doing, but entered into complicated agreements with the men and women they healed.[3] Elizabeth Cohen, Felippo de Vivo, and Patrick Wallis, to name only a few other scholars, have pointed to still other veins of archival material, especially Inquisitorial dossiers, as treasuries of information about the everyday operations of medicine at points of contact that Pamela Smith calls "trading zones," that is, both physical places and cultural spaces in which social and professional categories overlapped, making exchange and even collaboration possible.[4] These scholars have illuminated the varied functions and clientele of apothecary shops, pharmacists' strategies for holding their own in the fiercely competitive marketplace of medical and pharmaceutical knowledge, the hazy boundaries between "public" and "private" in the early-modern workforce, and the increasing commercialization of medicine.

Yet court records show us the past in a fractured mirror of crisis, which already presents an analytical problem if our question concerns the quotidian but becomes a major obstacle if we want to know about medical practitioners' everyday encounters specifically with literature and humanistic culture—beyond their ownership of prohibited books. One might assume that correspondence would be the best place to look, but the surviving letters of physicians, as Nancy Siraisi has shown, tend to be medical *consilia* by another name, intended to represent the ideals of their profession and not to divulge the details of an average day.[5] One turns, then, to the diary, that great desideratum of history. While far more difficult to find than court battles, *ricordi* ranging from extensive reminiscences to laconic account books do exist. What if we were to examine them less for what they might tell us about medical culture and more with what they could tell us about literary culture?

This chapter finds the literary in a set of such household records, two hitherto unexplored manuscript account books that Alberto Rini compiled over the course of his long life.[6] Ledgers more than family histories,

Rini nonetheless made room in their pages to record his cultural priorities and activities. A younger colleague of Nicolò Massa and Francesco Longo, Alberto Rini shows us an ordinary physician's cultural life. We have already made use of a few of his observations in previous chapters. It is time now to consider Rini's remarks in their own right.

Rini's observations do occasionally reveal his experiences of medicine, for instance, his passion for collecting recipes, but these notebooks yield less information about his specific line of work than about his and his family's accumulation of honor outside the world of healing. Alberto Rini's father, Benedetto, had also been a physician and began the family's tradition of punctilious keeping of accounts. Alberto followed his father professionally and in his careful attention to domestic economy. Under Alberto's stewardship, however, the Rini account books also became something closer to diaries, even if space constraints and generic conventions alike made them less discursive than we would expect a diary to be. Rini terms his account books "daily memoranda" *(giornali)* and while his entries are sometimes only a few words, taken as a whole the volumes provide a complex firsthand account of family, literary, and civic life during the last half of the sixteenth century. This lively and sharp-witted physician shared much with the category of Italian writers whom Armando Petrucci has wryly if genially termed "free literates," meaning men and women from the thirteenth century onward who read and wrote in the vernacular "apart from any precise social functions or constricting juridical obligations" and with a certain gusto, simply because they could.[7] A free literate in his approach, even if his university degrees would have enabled other forms of writing, Rini used his registers to record matters small and great, from grocery bills to his scholarly activities and the honors conferred on his family members.

Along the way, Rini also discussed the major events taking place in La Serenissima and throughout the peninsula with a spirit and level of attention that attest to his self-awareness as a citizen. While far more evidence than Rini's notes would be needed to make a case for an emergence of modern notions of citizenship in early-modern Venice, the question would be worth pursuing. Rini, a commoner with no immediate connection to the business of governance, exhibits both a fascination with high politics and a sense of authorization to comment on Venice's ruling elite no less than the people closest to him. This keen observer felt he had a stake in most everything.

Yet Rini's primary objective remained chronicling his life and his family—and that in itself is surprising, given our assumptions about the forms of family history on the ground in Venice in his era. James Grubb has argued that Venetians, unlike Florentines, did not keep *ricordanze.*[8] Attributing the comparative lack of examples to Venetians' closed patriciate, Grubb contends that the families most likely to have left *ricordanze*—especially new patrician families seeking to solidify and ornament their lineage with histories and claims to nobility—did not exist in Venice. Venetian patriciate itself, he also observes, had little need to record their family histories; they were already inscribed in the *libro d'oro* and could also rely on civic chroniclers, as well as humanist historians, to memorialize them. Venetian sources explicitly labeled *ricordanze, ricordi,* or even *libri di famiglia* (Barbaro's famous treatise aside) are exceptional. Yet, as I have been contending, we do well to consider early-modern archival sources as potential sites in which multiple genres might emerge and converge. While not family histories as such, many of the testaments we have analyzed and, as we will see here, account books, also left their creators room to remember their families, together with their literal and literary possessions. In pointing to the polyvalence of our sources, I build on Matthew Lundin's argument about the fundamentally experimental and inchoate nature of early-modern writing, certainly outside the context of formal academic or humanist compositions, and especially in forms of self-writing—what Lundin calls "paper memory."[9] Lundin's principal case study, the Cologne lawyer Hermann Weinsberg, bequeathed to his heirs nearly seven thousand pages of writing about himself and his forebears, as well as a voluminous testament and his lengthy exegesis of that document. Rini only left two notebooks, but we nonetheless find a similar interplay of journalistic reportage, sweeping family history, self-promotion and self-abnegation, and the partial appropriation of diverse literary styles ranging from poetry to spiritual autobiography. Indeed, we have occasion to make comparisons with Weinsberg at several points hereafter.

One point of comparison emerges at the outset: the impetus to record-keeping that bachelorhood may have provided. Like Weinsberg, Rini may have kept such careful records, in part, because he lacked legitimate bodily heirs. For individuals who did not have children to succeed them, posterity took on a peculiar significance.[10] Heirs required extensive management, but their existence offered some assurance that the memory of the parent and the family group would persist. For men and women like Weinsberg and Rini, posterity required active construction. Both Alberto Rini and his brother Scipione, in fact, lacked bodily heirs. None of the Rini family documents, including wills, mention spouses for either man, though they may both have had wives who died young. And of course the Rini brothers may have fathered illegitimate children. It seems as if Alberto had done so at least once, because in 1559 he recorded the death of "my daughter Isabella" *(Isabella mia figliuola),* noting that she had been ill for thirteen days.[11] In 1578, Alberto also sent a Roman breviary to a girl whom he termed his "little daughter" *(mia figliuolin),* who was living in the town of Sebenico.[12] The following year, he sent a painted chest to the same town, noting that the gift was for his *figlioccia* or goddaughter.[13] Given the different terms that Rini uses, it may be that in both cases (but particularly in the second) the girls were his illegitimate daughters or goddaughters of whom he was especially fond. In any event, Alberto Rini never mentions having a wife or an heir. And Scipione left everything to Alberto, meaning that Scipione, too, had not provided the family with an addition to its biological line. Yet the Rini brothers contributed to the family's posterity through their cultural attainments, if not through their children.

We have already seen that Rini bought books like a humanist. Now we can delve into details concerning his library, while considering Rini's journals more broadly as sites where this reader and collector turned chronicler. These records reveal Rini's eye both to civic history and to family memory. He made careful note of the elections of doges and popes, as well as the births, marriages, and deaths of family members and civic icons, but he gave equal attention and indeed very similar descriptions to even very humble personal and familial triumphs and losses. When Doge Pasquale Cicogna died, for instance, Rini remarked in an entry dated April 12, 1595, that "His Most Serene Highness . . . passed to the other life at approximately two o'clock this afternoon, having served as doge nine years, seven months and fifteen days. On Wednesday we learned that he had died and on Friday his funeral was held at the Church of Santi Giovanni e Paolo. His Excellency messer Enea Piccolomini, a public lecturer here in Venice, gave the funerary oration; thereafter the corpse was carried to the Croceri for burial."[14] The same attention to detail, and to the importance of the funerary orator, characterized Rini's approach even to the passing of a family pet. "Our dog Satin died today at four o'clock in the afternoon," Rini noted on August 3, 1560. "We buried him in the courtyard under the jasmine topiary near the laurel. Marina [our maid] gave the eulogy."[15]

Account books cover a wide range of topics, but as we examine Rini's we find that his observations cohere around the central concerns of individuals seeking cultural legitimacy. He noted his purchases of cheese, but he also inscribed the moments and possessions that showcased his and his family's greater achievements. Rini became most attentive to journalizing when he or another family member extended their competencies or networks beyond the world of medicine.

EXPANDING THE RINI FAMILY'S CULTURAL HORIZONS

The daily memoranda of Alberto Rini accentuate family members' acquisition of intellectual credentials and civic honor. For Rini, as for so many others, these two qualities sustained each other. Rini emphasizes his brother's university degrees. Yet in almost the same breath he records the family's networking and the gifts that he and other kin sent to patricians, senior colleagues, and even humanists to strengthen, enhance, and expand those networks.

Everything had resonance for Alberto Rini, but especially if it involved the acquisition of knowledge or honor. In 1559, Alberto paid twenty-six ducats (about 35 percent of his annual income) for the doctorate in medicine at Padua that his elder brother, Fabrizio, was about to take and thereafter Fabrizio's entrance fees at the Paduan College of Physicians. In that same year, Alberto paid for his other brother Scipione's doctorate in law, also taken at Padua. As we have seen several times, families with social ambitions hoped to send children to university. Artisan fathers aimed to get one son a medical degree and fathers with medical degrees to have one son at law. Even as a relatively young man, with a living father, Alberto Rini had already taken the role of family record keeper and even exerted a distinctly paternal role in funding his brothers' university studies. These exertions earned Alberto special recognition from his father: Benedetto bequeathed to Alberto special legacies in his will, including custodianship of his most prized possession, a gorgeous illuminated herbal, explicitly because Alberto had already shown himself to be devoted to the family's honor, much of it rooted in connection to the universities.[16]

Rini supported his brothers' progress toward university degrees and tracked each step these credentials enabled the young men to take toward inner-circle belonging among Venice's cultural and social elite. Here was another physician who knew the complex calculus of cultural legitimacy. Rini recorded his family members' achievements and the favors they received from their social superiors. He also signaled relatives' increasing involvement in the activities of the civic elite by tracking notable events in the lives of patricians to whom the Rini had formed some connection, however tenuous.

It was with particular relish that Alberto recorded his brother Scipione's increasing civic prominence. Scipione had advanced the family beyond the ranks of physicians to that of lawyers, and Alberto eagerly noted the honors Scipione began to accumulate. In 1566, Scipione joined Antonio Piran (another lawyer) as joint godfather to the son of an acquaintance. That same year the Venetian governor of Candia, Zuanne Mocenigo, favored Scipione with a gift basket that included wine, cheese, pastries, and herbs. In 1588, Scipione stood as godfather for twin boys, Alvise and Antonio, born to the patrician Valaresso family. "On the day of Epiphany, at dawn (more or less)," Alberto excitedly reports, "two male infants were born at the same time to The Most Illustrious Lady Elisabetta Miani, wife of The Most Illustrious Lord Zaccharia Valaresso, son of The Most Illustrious Alvise, who is also our neighbor. And on the 12th of that month both of the boys were baptized in the Church of San Provolo, with The Reverend messer Giacomo Sasso, our priest, officiating. There were twenty-two godfathers present, among them my brother messer Scipione, who also held the twins."[17] Alberto Rini's use of possessives marked his participation and that of the whole family in the compliment paid to Scipione in being chosen as a godfather for the Valaresso twins. Alvise Valaresso, Alberto specifies, was "our" neighbor and the priest was "our" priest. Possibly with an eye to the comprehension of future readers, Rini also adds details that would have been unnecessary in a private record intended only for his own use, for example, that Scipione was his brother and that he warranted the title "messer." In the same spirit, Rini emphasized in 1590 that Scipione was the sole godfather of Franceschina Laura Marcello, daughter of another patrician, Lorenzo di Bartolomeo Marcello.[18]

Scipione's entrance in 1588 into the Scuola Grande di San Marco, Venice's preeminent confraternity, elicited one of Alberto's most loquacious entries. Alberto had himself become a brother there, but never recorded that moment. Scipione's achievement, by contrast, warranted special mention. Likely because Scipione had his degree in law, he had been earmarked as the heir responsible for advancing the Rinis in the city. Membership in the Scuola Grande di San Marco promised good results in that line. "I note here that today messer Scipione my brother was voted into the Scuola of San Marco," Alberto announces. "This was thanks to the fact that Scipione had been one of the executors for the late messer Piero Venier. [Scipione] had eighteen ballots in his favor, and eight against him. I was one of the eighteen in favor, along with [Venier's other executors] messer Bartolomeo Moro the lawyer, messer Marco Zon, messer Hieronimo di Franceschi and messer Andrea Dardani . . . as well as messer Cesare Ziliol and messer Marc'Antonio Gerardo."[19] Alberto was fond of his brother, but Scipione's successes also enhanced the prestige of the family.

The achievements of extended kin and friends also redounded to the honor of the Rinis and thus earned a place in Alberto's journals. He recorded, for instance, that a family friend, Marc'Antonio Calafado, had been admitted to the Scuola Grande di San Marco in 1590, "thanks to the

Clarissimo Francesco Gerardo, Secretary of the Council of Ten." This Secretary Gerardo had seen to it that Calafado, though he was only artisan rank (his title is "mistro"), joined the sodality *gratis,* that is, without the usual dues. Secretary Gerardo did Calafado this extraordinary favor, Rini observes, "on our behalf."[20] Rini had two particular reasons to be pleased about his friend Calafado's advancement: Calafado's success proved that Rini's patronage networks were working well, and this circumstance also allowed Rini to extend the godfather role that he had already been playing for the Calafado family. Three years before Marc'Antonio Calafado's acceptance into the Scuola, a man called Tomaso Calafado had been accepted into the Scuola free of charge, once again through the good offices of Secretary Gerardo. This Tomaso Calafado, Rini specifies, was "one of my godsons."[21]

Nor did Rini neglect the importance of female kin in family advancement: He expressed considerable pleasure whenever his female relatives married well. In 1594, he recorded (twice) the wedding of "Her Magnificence Bortolamia de Ca' de Piero," the daughter of Rini's cousin Gerolemo Piero, to a certain Gadi Gadi "a gentleman from Forlì and a very rich merchant." In his first note, Rini wishes his second cousin (whom he calls his "niece") happiness and good fortune. In an additional note, dated a week later, he records further details about the wedding, especially that Bortolamia brought to the marriage a dowry of more than six thousand ducats.[22] Rini tracked the dowries of patrician women from families with which he had some acquaintance, including his note about the 1594 wedding of His Magnificence Giulio Gerardo to Helena, daughter of Angelo dalla Vedova, that the bride had been given an eighteen-thousand-ducat dowry.[23]

Once again, we see the outlines of a Venetian family's rise to moderate stature by way of the university and through the cultivation of friendship and patronage networks. While starting off with a father in the medical field helped, Rini shows us the considerable effort required to move beyond that professional level. In his own way, Rini's notations concerning his family's expanding cultural horizons remind us of how much work was left to be done, even by a family with university graduates, if they aimed for more prestige.

Rini's preoccupation with the place of his kin on the social map of Venice also expressed itself in a literary way, his keen interest in family history as a genre. Late in his life (1594), Alberto visited a chapel at the Crociere in search of information about his paternal grandfather and namesake. He was pleased to find there a series of relief portraits, a roll call (circa 1499) of "important men in the silk weaving craft," among them the elder Alberto Rini.[24] These guild-commissioned portraits documented the steady progress of Rini's family, from his paternal grandfather, who earned an honorable place in the mercantile world, to Rini himself and even more so his brother Scipione, men who now interacted regularly with members of the patriciate. The same interest in family history informed Alberto's records of all the births and deaths in the family of his maternal grandfather, Zuanne Bonaldi.[25]

As the years wore on, Rini's predilection for family history inspired him to purchase books in the genre of biography, especially those concerning the nobility. At a similar stage of life, the Cologne lawyer Hermann Weinsberg had begun to think of lineage in expansive ways, including the invention of an ancient and noble genealogy, complete with fictitious coat of arms, for his artisanal forebears.[26] Rini did not approach lineage with quite this much creativity, but he read and circulated among friends texts helpful for imagining a style of life to which future members of the Rini family might become accustomed. During the last decade of his life (1584-1599), Rini often noted the purchase of biographies of Italian notables, which he sometimes also offered as gifts to patricians whom he hoped to cultivate.

In a manner typical of early-modern Europeans, this Venetian physician maintained his social networks through gift exchange.[27] In general, Rini, like others, tended to make gifts of objects that signaled his own status and complimented his recipients. As he was an educated man and learning ranked so high in the cultural priorities of the day, Rini presented friends, patrons, or especially important colleagues with books or manuscripts. In 1584, he lent to the nobleman Luc'Antonio Giunti a chronicle that Rini himself had transcribed "of the exploits of the nobility, in arms and otherwise."[28] Deepening his familiarity with the genre, perhaps with a thought of transcribing other works to use as gifts to noblemen, Rini would subsequently purchase for himself Paolo Giovio's encyclopedia of accomplishment, *De viris illustribus,* as well as a book on the origin of the Italian nobility, and a who's who of Genoese celebrities. In 1597, he ingratiated himself with "His Magnificence, Signor Giulio Gerardo," who at the time served as the Venetian ambassador in Florence, by sending Gerardo an elaborate manuscript "on nobility, copied by messer Lorenzo the Tuscan" for which Rini had paid twelve lire. This manuscript cost Rini six times what he spent on cheese in a month, and more than seven times his monthly expenditure for oil. Even the two most expensive volumes that he purchased for himself, a deluxe hardback edition of Francesco Panigarola's sermons and a treatise on surgery by Alvise Bognolo della Croce, each cost roughly half of what he paid for the presentation manuscript on the Italian nobility that he sent to Gerardo. Most of Rini's personal book expenditures hovered between sixteen soldi for unbound books and one lira twelve soldi for bound copies. Clearly Rini meant to cultivate this Venetian statesman, to whom he also loaned travel narratives and accounts of the Spanish and Neapolitan courts.[29]

Like many cultured people, then, Rini knew how to use literary material as the currency of friendship. But even gifts of comestibles tended to cement his bonds with other learned men. In 1581, for instance, Rini sent large wheels of pecorino cheese to the lawyer Giovanni Battista Bartoli and to the physician Belisario Gadaldino.[30] Rini did especially well to ingratiate himself with Gadaldino, a son of the celebrated physician-humanist Agostino Gadaldino, who had already earned prominence on his own merits. Belisario Gadaldino served two terms as prior of the College, 1578–1579 and 1580–1581, the same year he found himself the recipient of Rini's wheel of pecorino.[31] Gadaldino's erudition earned significant notice as well; he was called on more often than any other College member to give the Latin orations at colleagues' funerals. In 1573, Gadaldino orated for Andrea Baranzon and Nicolò Tinto. In 1576, he marked the passing of Gerolemo Grataruol. And on September 13, 1577, Gadaldino enjoyed the signal honor of being one of three orators chosen for the lavish three-stage funeral of the renowned physician and scholar Tomaso Filologo of Ravenna, whom the College of Venice had poached years previously and with much fanfare from his post at Padua.[32] As we have seen, Gadaldino was also a prominent member of the editorial team who brought Vettore Trincavella's collected works to press. In his vita of Trincavella, Lorenzo Marucini celebrates Gadaldino, alongside Gerolemo Mercuriale, as Trincavella's student and editor.[33] In this same edition, Gadaldino performed the role of publicist, writing a lengthy epistle to the reader that constitutes an apologia for medicine as a liberal art and a service to the common good.[34]

Like Francesco Longo, despite his learning and connections to the republic of letters, Rini does not seem to have published any compositions. Unlike Longo, however, Rini actively maintained connections to the literary world, partly in service to his father's legacy. Alberto's father, Benedetto, made one important contribution to medical theory, a treatise on syphilis, which Alvise Luisin included in his monumental compendium of syphilis tracts, *De morbo gallico* (1566–1567).[35] Luisin also enlisted Alberto's brother, the physician Fabrizio Rini, to rededicate Benedetto Rini's treatise to Antonio Cauco, then archbishop of Corcyra.[36] In the same year that *De morbo gallico* emerged from the press, Luisin also gave the funeral oration for Benedetto Rini to an audience of "nearly all the physicians" of the College.[37] Luisin was most likely Benedetto Rini's protégé. Students often gave the funerary orations for their teachers, as Domenico Castelli had done for

Vettore Trincavella. In these orations, the student played a filial role as well, because kinship was the primary language for signifying close relationships of many kinds, not least of them academic. Castelli represented his relationship to Trincavella as that of a son to a father. "How could I ever with dry eyes gaze upon him, dead, lying here in the middle of the church?" Castelli asked the other mourners. "Or should I witness without a deep groan the exequies of a teacher who behaved so lovingly toward me—he who always treated me like a son and in whose methods and expertise I was trained, so to speak, from childhood?"[38] In Alvise Luisin, who likely played a similar role as Benedetto Rini's discursive son, Alberto Rini also had a discursive brother with a sturdy publication record, and one who helped commemorate Benedetto Rini's accomplishments.

Even if Alberto Rini did not use his connections in the world of letters to publish, his loose affiliation with learned circles enhanced his private intellectual life. Diana Robin has furnished us with a brilliant image of the proto-salons of the Cinquecento, with their intricate webs of intellectual and textual exchange made visible in multiple print publications, but we are less clear-sighted about those who did not publish.[39] While no evidence survives that Rini ever came forward as an author in his own right, his journals nonetheless show us, if not quite the regular and immediate rewards of participation in a salon, at least evidence that contact with literati fueled his own literary pursuits and sometimes supplied him with much-needed books and manuscripts. The networks he continued and extended, and which his gift giving sustained, enhanced the family's cultural legitimacy in the aggregate even as they furthered Rini's own reading and writing projects.

A BIBLIOPHILE AND COPYIST

Alberto Rini had a rich intellectual life. He collected books and preserved those already acquired by his family members. He eagerly transcribed chronicles and sermons. He also observed and described his world, even if in few words. In imagining the contours of Nicolò Massa's library, we had occasion to discuss the Rini library and Alberto's acquisitions in a general way; here we will consider its contents in more detail. But Rini's journals show that this reader also used his acquisitions as models. After looking more closely through his library, we will see Rini not only buying and circulating texts but also drawing a measure of authorial inspiration from them.

The custodian of a library that ultimately encompassed, considering his own additions, five hundred volumes, Rini had a wealth of reading material. As we have already learned, by the time the Rini household and books were inventoried (1604, several years after Alberto's death), the collection constituted a predominantly literary library. He may have given a considerable collection of medical books as gifts to colleagues or students, but the library that remained to posterity was the library of a humanist more than a physician. We recall that only 4 percent of the collection pertained to medicine, if we include the Rini holdings in the Aristotelian corpus, and only 2 percent if we count Aristotle instead as ancient literature. The collection clustered around three major areas: ancient literature (74 volumes; 88 if we include Aristotle); modern humanist epistles, history, biography, and poetry (161 volumes); and theology (82 volumes). But the library also encompassed a significant number of reference works (twenty-four volumes, predominantly dictionaries, grammars, and guides to style), and even a fair representation of drama and music (six modern plays and fifteen songbooks). In other words, this library represented in a high degree the major cultural currents of the day.

This literary conservator, circulator, and collector had myriad interests and an extensive library through which to pursue them, but he naturally had his preferences. Those preferences had only the most tangential connection to his occupation. To judge by the texts he made a special effort to transcribe in his own hand, Rini's particular interests lay in chronicles and sermons.

Many, if by no means all, medieval scholars represented copying texts as an honorable activity that engaged the mind and, in the case of religious material, conferred spiritual benefits. By the seventeenth century, while some scholars still upheld these sentiments, many disparaged copying, transcribing, and sometimes even note-taking as passive and tedious mechanical labor.[40] In Rini's lifetime both positions had their adherents, but his contemporaries were still more inclined than their successors would be to adopt the position of a Petrarch, or for that matter a Jesuit instructor, that in the case of truly important texts, the intellectual should serve as their own scribe, abbreviator, or note taker—in part to avoid the errors of professional copyists but more importantly to fix the material more effectively in their minds.

In his first journal, Rini noted that he had loaned to a Zuanne Spinelli a chronicle that Rini had written in his own hand.[41] Rini's second journal shows him busy transcribing a wide assortment of chronicles and histories throughout the 1580s and 1590s. Of particular interest was Rini's work in 1581 and 1582, the years in which he avidly copied the chronicles of Doge Andrea Dandolo (d. 1354). Rini had borrowed manuscript redactions of these texts from the humanist historian Paolo Ramusio.[42] Over the next few months, Rini ran several times to the printer's shop for ink and new notebooks, "in which to copy Dandolo's chronicle."[43] These Latin chronicles, known as the *Chronica brevis* and *Chronica per extensum descripta*, constituted foundational texts in Venetian political philosophy. Dandolo was himself the archetypal Renaissance doge; he had taken his law degree from the University of Padua, was a friend of Petrarch, and a patron of the arts.[44] Rini's interest in Dandolo, evident in the months he devoted to transcribing the text, underscores again his interests well outside his occupational field. In the later 1580s, these interests would extend to transcribing the history of Venice written by Giovanni Giacomo Caroldo, secretary of the Council of Ten. In this case, Rini borrowed the original text from Caroldo's nephew Nicolò.[45]

These projects in the genre of chronicles illustrate Rini's special interest in history, an interest that connects him both to the mainstream of the contemporary republic of letters and, as Nancy Siraisi has shown, to the extracurricular literary interest most commonly found among members of the medical profession.[46] This passion also underscores Rini's alignment with and active use of his family's library. The Rini household inventory lists ninety-three books that belonged in the genre of history, if we count both ancient and humanist historical writing, as well as all the subgenres of chronicle, chronology, biography, and descriptions of antiquities, as well as local and "world" histories.[47] In other words, historical material constituted nearly 19 percent of this large collection. Rini's concern with transcribing the Dandolo manuscript, moreover, signals an at least provisionally humanist mode of working; he returned to the source. Venetian presses churned out myriad histories of the city, most of which borrowed heavily from Dandolo and other earlier chronicles. Rini, however, insisted on reading Dandolo in the original. While personal or civic interest surely constituted part of his motivation, this project also accentuated and strengthened his connections in a material way to the world of letters.

Rini's transcription of Dandolo made him new friends in humanist places. By borrowing the Dandolo manuscript from Paolo Ramusio, Rini acted, in the terms Brian Maxson has given us, as a "social humanist"—someone who may not have published, but who engaged in correspondence and other forms of exchange with humanists who did.[48] Ramusio was a noted scholar and collector, whom the celebrated physician-historian Gerolemo Mercuriale praised as "an excellent man and most studious of good letters and all beautiful things."[49] Rini cultivated his connection to Ramusio over the course of decades.

The link between the Rini family and Ramusio persisted through at least the 1580s. Several years after Alberto Rini borrowed Dandolo's chronicles,

Ramusio witnessed the will of Scipione Rini.[50] This service attested to Ramusio's willingness to occupy the role of extended kin. Witnessing was not the sort of function you would, or from a legal standpoint could, perform unless you considered yourself a close colleague or family friend. Alberto Rini also notes in February of 1588 that Ramusio had performed another friendly service for him, procuring a luxurious office of the Madonna. Rini describes this text with an attention to detail he seldom accords even to his other bibliographic acquisitions. Usually Rini notes the book's author or title and sometimes the publisher, if it was one of the city's more prestigious presses. He noted, for instance, that he bought a collection of ancient Roman imperial biographies including Nerva, Trajan, and Hadrian from the city's premier publishing house of Aldus Manutius.[51] Describing the office of the Madonna procured by one of Venice's literary celebrities, however, Rini took even more time to narrate the acquisition: "I had, thanks to His Magnificence Signore Paolo Ramusio, a little office of the Madonna, sent to me from France by Ramusio's son Signore Gerolemo, who was a royal secretary to the Most Christian King of France along with the Illustrious Signore Zuanne Dolfin; the office was printed in Antwerp in 1586 and is covered in reddish leather with a golden band around it."[52] Rini's unusually detailed description of this transaction suggests that the extended humanist networks who had brought this item to his library were, in his mind, nearly as valuable as the book itself; certainly, they were as noteworthy.

In addition to being attuned to Dandolo, Rini was an avid transcriber of sermons, another passion that had little direct bearing on his profession but enriched his intellectual, literary, and presumably spiritual life. Beginning in 1584, Rini began retranscribing his father's copies of the sermons of Cardinal Bertano.[53] Ann Blair has suggested that the habitus of transcription and copying tended to move through families, both as a practice and through the bequests of such volumes, a suggestion for which the Rini furnish supplementary evidence.[54] Continuing this practice into the 1590s, Rini ultimately began to record the new sermons he had attended, as we learn from his regular expenditures of ten soldi for "copybooks for writing down the sermons."[55] On one occasion, Rini was able once again to use his writing as a gift (this time of thanks) to recognize Nicolò Caroldo's generosity in lending him his uncle's history of Venice. Rini gave to Caroldo "twenty copybooks of the sermons of the Reverend Brisighella, to send to the Reverend Giacomo di Conti, a monk at San Michele in Padua."[56]

Even in the tight space of his account book, Rini's tiny merchant hand found room to indicate his participation in Venice's cultural life at large. He proved his connection to the literary world as he busied himself not only buying books but investing the time and effort into copying manuscripts. This physician, like the others we have met, had a good deal of connection to other forms of engagement in his immediate socioprofessional world. His activities and interests extended not only to moving in humanist friendship networks but also engaging with the market in recipes and secrets. Much as he bought and preserved books of different sorts, so he sought solutions to logistical and health problems from as wide a variety of sources as did most of his contemporaries. Let us consider what he tells us of this marketplace before turning to his most creative work as an observer and chronicler.

RINI AND THE WORLD OF SECRETS

Pamela Smith, William Eamon, and many others have stressed the intersections of literary and manual knowledge in early-modern scientific communities. Eamon, in particular, has pointed to the trade in secrets and recipes as a realm in which we see the exchange of men and women from different backgrounds and the hybridization of literary and experimental practices.[57] Rini's passion for recording useful recipes and secret remedies, no less than his penchant for histories, chronicles, and sermons, proved him to be a man of his era.

Given his reading and writing projects, it is not surprising that Rini invested regularly in paper and ink; however, given his limited resources, it is also not surprising that he tried his hand at making ink at home.[58] Rini sometimes paid the steep price of ten soldi for a particularly good ink from a bookseller near the Piazza San Marco. At other times, he settled for less luxurious brands.[59] One senses that poor ink quality (whatever the price) was a regular source of frustration for Rini, who in 1584 eagerly transcribed a recipe from his friend Domenico a Salis for making "a very black and excellent ink" at home—a recipe that involved bringing a combination of gum arabic, vitriol, gall, and a sturdy white wine to a boil twice, after which "it will be done and will turn out perfectly."[60] It seems that Rini was initially happy with the results and pursued do-it-yourself ink making for a few years, but he ultimately returned to buying his ink.

Rini's ink project exemplifies the energy with which he directed his collector's instincts and his graphomania to gathering recipes. To readers of Deborah Harkness's splendid account of the trade in medical and scientific knowledge among men and women from many different backgrounds in Elizabethan London, it may seem natural that an Italian physician of the same era should also have busied himself in collecting recipes and "secrets."[61] But technically speaking learned physicians like Rini were supposed to distance themselves from anything akin to the cures peddled by "empirics." This derogatory category sometimes encompassed surgeons and pharmacists, practitioners with licenses but usually no formal university training, as well as "wise" men and women termed *ciarlatani* (charlatans) who could be found in every neighborhood. At the least, trading in recipes and medical secrets brought the physician from his tidy Galenic library into the mucky streets of the medical marketplace.

Early in 1586, Rini had found a plague remedy in the form of a "garlic sauce to make during times of plague" *(agliata da fare in tempo di peste),* which had been used, he says, by a certain "Abbot of Saccolongo." This recipe was for what we now call *pesto basilico:* fresh basil, garlic, and nuts ground together to form a paste. While we put the sauce on hot pasta on all occasions, according to Rini it should be eaten cold and on its own when plague strikes.[62] Rini had lived through two waves of plague before he found this recipe, so it cannot have been the only preventative medicine available. At least equally effective was fleeing the city as quickly as possible after the plague hit, which is what Alberto and Scipione did late in 1574–1575. We learn of the Rinis' absence from Venice during the calamity from Alberto's explanation for the gap in his recordkeeping. "I note here that there have not been any records of expenses [of late]," he explains, "because we've found ourselves out of town, owing to the death and pestilence that have been in the city of Venice for seven months without abatement." Rini also included in his notebook the "passport" out of the city granted by the *Provveditori sopra la sanità* to his brother Scipione and Scipione's maid on September 7, 1576. This passport asserted that none of them exhibited any signs of the "mal contagioso," attesting that even a month after the plague had left the city, fear remained.[63]

Rini's other recipes promised remedies for more common maladies including flatulence, worms, and backaches that called for a variety of herbs, spices, and common house-and-garden ingredients. A drink made of nutmeg, ginger, clove, and oregano promised relief from flatulence. A laurel-based unguent might be used to drive out worms, and another unguent, formed of marjoram, violets, a woman's breast milk, and egg whites, would soothe backaches.[64] As a regular part of their work, physicians offered broadly conceived dietary advice to their patients (generally to eat more or less food, or drink more or less wine) as a means to recalibrate their Galenic humoral imbalances. Rini does not situate these remedies in this framework; rather, he treats the recipes *in themselves* as specific remedies for particular ailments. In so doing, he may reveal himself to have been among the minority of sixteenth-century physicians who took Paracelsus's view of illness, conceiving of diseases as entities that required specific chemical treatments instead of the dietary and life advice—and bleeding—that other physicians advised. At all events, Rini seems to have been as eager for "empirical" relief as his contemporaries were.

Rini must have recognized the potential professional taboo of his recipes and secrets, because he occludes his sources in these cases, whereas he cited his informants and collaborators punctiliously in case of literary endeavors. Rini credited his recipe for *pesto basilico,* as we have seen, to an unidentifiable "abbot." The flatulence cure has no attribution. Rini specifies that he got the remedy for worms from someone from the "da Rio" family who was dead (being noted as "q" or quondam in the entry). Rini never provides a given name, offering instead a string of honorifics "the Magnificent," "His Excellency," and the two letters *D* and *R,* which probably indicate "Domino" (Lord) and "Reverendo" (Reverend). The individual attributed was thus a patrician, a university graduate, and a cleric. But his surname Rio (meaning "canal") was more common in watery Venice than "Jones" is in Wales. And in any case, the author of the cure for worms was deceased and so unavailable for further questioning. Rini credited the recipe for backaches yet more laconically to a certain "MGM" (possibly "[Il] Magnifico Gerolemo Mercuriale").

One might argue that Rini, scribbling in narrow ledgers, simply abbreviated everything because of space constraints. When he wanted to emphasize his sources, however, he found room to do so. For instance, the reader finds Paolo Ramusio's name unabbreviated as the source of the Dandolo manuscripts. So, too, when a "recipe" had no healing value attached to it, he credited his source. For example, we have Rini's instructions for softening coriander seeds prior to using them in ordinary cooking, not a professional liability as it did not specifically involve a "cure." Accordingly, there was no reason for Rini not to note in this case that he had learned the coriander-preparation technique from "His Excellency, my colleague messer Gerolemo di Lodovici."[65]

Rini's collection of remedies and recipes constitutes rare glimpses into his experience of practical medicine. As a rule, these journals do not discuss his practice or any other form of his work in the medical marketplace. He did keep track of his father's earnings. And Rini also noted, during the plague crisis of 1576, "I set aside to give to the physician of our parish 3 lire 2 soldi."[66] Accordingly, we learn that Rini was not the physician of his parish and that, while exiting the city himself during the epidemic as many physicians did (indeed, were encouraged to do so, in order that they might live to serve the community thereafter), Rini nonetheless offered some financial support to the doctor responsible for tending the neighborhood.[67] He never mentions consultations with patients or fees received for medical work. Indeed, it seems that his most regular income derived from managing rental properties, as was true for many citizen-rank Venetians.[68]

We learn a bit more from Rini about the experience of medicine through his recording of the pharmaceuticals and procedures he sought when ill. Physician or not, Rini sought the full range of healing options to which most of his contemporaries subscribed. As Elizabeth Cohen, Mary Lindemann, David Gentilcore, and others have shown, when faced with a malady, people sought out multiple avenues of healing rather than any one type of practitioner or remedy.[69] Even those who might eschew the services of priests and cunning women still had recourse to an array of options, from household recipes to the spices and syrups on offer at apothecaries' shops, as well as the assistance of barber-surgeons and, if they could afford it, the advice of a university-trained physician. Rini, too, pursued different avenues of healing.

When home remedies proved insufficient, Rini turned to apothecaries. Finding himself indisposed one spring, and perhaps suffering more than usual on account of the rigors of the Lenten fast, Rini headed to the apothecary at the Sign of the Egg for some "medicinal spices."[70] On another occasion, he notes, he was suffering an excessive "humidity in my head" (possibly a sinus infection or migraine), and so he went to a different pharmacist in San Marco who was licensed to sell the "legno santo" ("holy wood" or guiac), a medicine made from a tree found in the Caribbean regularly administered to those who had contracted the pox (syphilis), but that was also used to treat other ailments.[71] For maladies that he deemed better served by stronger methods, Rini enlisted surgeons. It seems that Rini was troubled by gout. In 1581, he submitted himself twice to bleeding at the hands of "His Excellency, Sappia the surgeon."[72] While bleeding was ubiquitously administered for a host of different maladies, it is significant that Rini only notes having himself bled in this one instance. And this event is closely followed by a transcription of a remedy for gout that he attributes (vaguely, as always) to "a doctor named Costa, lecturer at Bologna."[73] In 1598, Rini needed another surgeon to help with a problem that might also have been related to gout, which wreaks such havoc on the lower body. Rini notes that he had dislocated one of his feet. This time, Rini went not to Sappia but to "His Excellency messer Antonio," who worked at the Sign of the Two Physicians.[74] And it seems that his friend, the surgeon Gerolemo di Lodovici, at least by the mid-1580s, occasionally served in this capacity. In one entry Rini refers to Lodovici as "our doctor" *(nostro medico)*.[75] This is the only reference that Rini makes that indicates consultations about his ailments. Yet, despite the fact he had more formal training than Lodovici, evidently he still sometimes felt it prudent to get a second opinion in his own case and felt it unethical to advise Scipione himself. By the 1590s, Rini also called on the services of "His Excellency, Benedetto Gaio," whom he termed "our doctor."[76]

Is there a "medical perspective" in Rini's journals? While there are certainly indications of his status, one of the intriguing things about these journals is that they once again show us a physician involved in almost anything but medical theory or practice. The reader has no trouble discerning that Rini was a physician. Especially in his first journal (1557–1574) Rini kept track of doctors' funerals, specifying that these men were his colleagues. In addition to the record of Vettore Trincavella's funeral that we have already explored, we find notices of the passing of the physicians Gerolemo Boniperto from Novara and Maffeo dei Maffei.[77] Indeed, the first journal is closer to a necrology of relatives and colleagues, with some expense records, than the second journal (1574–1599), which is considerably more discursive. Other than attending to his colleagues' deaths, however, Rini does not reflect on the profession of medicine as such or mention the activities of the College. And even when the topic of plague emerges in 1576, Rini makes only general observations of the sort that most of his contemporaries could have made. "I note here," Rini wrote on April 25, 1576, "that today the convent of San Zaccharia was closed, because one of the nuns died and the physicians suspect that the cause of death was plague. I note this as a memorandum. May Lord God, in his divine mercy, not allow that scourge to proceed farther."[78] Rini did not venture his own theories or observations. He only hoped, with the rest of the city, for divine mercy.

Admittedly, whenever anyone died, whether close family or public figures, Rini specified the cause of death. In his attention to maladies, we may see something of Rini's professional deformity.[79] On March 10, 1582, Rini recorded the death of his cousin Gerolemo di Pietro, explaining that Gerolemo "had been ill for approximately two years from consumption."[80] Pope Pius IV got a similar treatment. Rini noted that the pontiff "died on Sunday at ten o'clock at night, from colic."[81] Rini's comments on the death of his brother Scipione were understandably freighted with far more emotion than these other notices, but he did still include the medical problem involved. "Jesus, Mary," Alberto writes, "On this day 14 November 1590, I, Alberto, here note that today my dearest and sweetest brother messer Scipione passed from this to the other life. May our Lord God have mercy on his soul. His last illness was a powerful apoplectic fit, which ended his life in the space of nine hours. The fit began midmorning and lasted until the Ave Maria this evening, when he closed his eyes in eternal sleep."[82] Physicians may have been even closer than their contemporaries were to disease and death, which were in any case a part of everyone's daily experience in early-modern Europe, but they still suffered in the encounter. And medical doctors seem to have felt, naturally enough, an acute frustration when the victims were family. Nicolò Massa told readers of his treatise on contagious fevers that both his father and his brother had died from diseases in this category; he even notes that he had the ability to recognize the fever in his brother's case, although he had not yet become a physician.[83] Physicians, then, might be able to recognize diseases better than others and might be more inclined to specify them, but they were just as powerless as anyone else to help.

POETRY, ART, AND POLITICS

Rini sought refuge from the harsh vicissitudes of life in his reading, collecting, transcribing, engaging with humanists, and even experimenting with recipes. In turning to writing as a form of retreat, Rini engaged in a practice that Pierre Hadot has shown to be characteristic of that paradigmatic philosopher-in-the-world, Marcus Aurelius.[84] Rini may or may not have consciously modeled himself or his writing on this ancient Roman precedent. No editions of the *Meditations* appear in the inventory of the Rini library (and several redactions of Marcus's biography and writings were available), but Scipione Rini's will names as one of his principal heirs a nephew who in fact bore the name Marco Aurelio; so, this model of Stoicism was certainly well known to the family.[85] And when Rini turned, however briefly, to poetic composition, he did so on a Stoic theme much in keeping with the sentiments of his nephew's imperial namesake. At all events, Rini's journals embed a number of distinct literary genres even if the notebooks left little room to develop them at any length. We see Rini testing out poetry, but also describing natural catastrophes and their casualties; he chronicled political events as well. Even if Rini's journals, with all their entries no more than a few sentences and usually only a few words, pale in comparison to the seven thousand pages of recollections and ruminations left by his contemporary Hermann Weinsberg, nonetheless Rini, in his own way, wrote his world.

Let us consider first Rini's poetry. In this experiment, Rini tried his hand at humanist writing—literally. In a collection of undated memoranda at the end of his first journal, Rini twice inscribed the same short poem. In one instance, he gave the poem a Latin title "Impotence, Necessity" *(impotentia, necessitas)*. While Rini usually wrote a cramped notarial hand, he attempted in these cases to write a calligraphic italic script, deeming it a more suitable medium for poetry. In this less practiced humanist hand, we find an epigram advocating stoic equilibrium:

> *Se al nostro mal il lagrimar giovasse,*
> *Sempre col pianto il duol tor si potrebbe,*
> *Et il pianto con or si comprarebbe.*
>
> If lamentation healed our wounds,
> Tears could always ease the pain,
> And gold would buy the tears.[86]

Rini repudiates self-pity. If surrendering to grief really did any good, he reasons, then we would be able to buy tears just like any other medicine. The only remedy, in the end, is to accept necessity. In his choice of neo-Stoicism as a mode, Rini, like Longo, echoed a distinct trend in the contemporary republic of letters. As Jason Saunders, Jill Kraye, Christopher Brooke, and others have demonstrated, while Stoic tenets interested scholastics and early Renaissance thinkers, it would be with Justus Lipsius that Christian or neo-Stoicism became a major element of humanist philosophy.[87] While Brooke's recent work emphasizes, rightly, the political dimension to neo-Stoicism, both Longo in his testaments and Rini in his experiment in poetry remind us that Stoicism had applications at home as much as it did in the forum. In this poem, too, Rini reminds us again of the model articulated by Hadot's Marcus Aurelius—especially the importance of concise, ruminative, and even repetitive writing as a retreat from the forum and "spiritual practice."[88]

Rini only tried the voice of the poet once, but he often assumed the role of the historical observer. In so doing, he practiced, in a miniature form, the modes of writing familiar to him from his reading and transcribing of chronicles and the deeds of the nobility. By far the most detailed of Rini's descriptions concerns the fire that struck the ducal palace in December 1577. Here was another disaster in his city, another crisis following closely upon the epidemic of plague. In rigorous detail, Rini recounts the progress of the conflagration as it made its way from a side street into the palace interior. He praises the coordinated efforts of fire brigades from the Arsenale, regular citizens, and divine mercy, which saved most of the newer wing of the palace and the nearby basilica of San Marco. Still, Rini's point is the magnitude of the disaster, which touched every part of the city. "The bells resounded from two in the afternoon to nearly midnight," he narrates. "The campanile at San Marco sounded and the bells of every church in every parish. Multitudes of patricians and armed citizens were immediately deputized to patrol the streets, marching day and night through the piazza, which was lit by an infinite number of torches and lights—and wax candles illuminated every balcony of every house, new and old. Nowhere in the annals of human memory has such a conflagration been recorded; it lasted until three o'clock in the morning."[89] Thanks to the timely intervention of Saint Mark, who could not countenance damage to his basilica, the winds quieted after threatening to spread from the palace to the church. Thanks to the "exemplary virtue and industry" of Venetian workmen, the fire itself was controlled before it spread to offices in the new wing of the ducal palace.[90] Emphasizing the valorous leadership of noblemen and the industry of commoners, Rini echoes tropes of historical writing dating back to antiquity that segregate the polity's virtues according to social station. He had read his histories and chronicles well.

The objects lost in the conflagration, however, bring Rini to a more distinctive lamentation that reveals once again his cultural priorities. In the whole narrative of the fire, what pained him most was the destruction of precious works of art and sculpture. "Both of the great halls in the ducal palace were completely burned," Rini laments. "And along with them, along with them ravishing paintings by Bellini and by Titian, and the ceiling murals. And the two colonnades fractured. And many of the marble columns supporting the balconies, which were exceptionally beautiful, collapsed."[91] Aesthetic casualties weighed most heavily on Rini's heart. And paintings were the most tragic losses, to judge by his phrasing. It was not just rooms and beautiful architectural ornamentation that perished, but "along with them, along with them" *(insieme, insieme)* works by two of Venice's great masters, Bellini and Titian.

Rini grieves as a connoisseur of art. While his journals only note a few aesthetic expenditures of his own, he did record the purchase of a painting of Cleopatra for one lira sixteen soldi in 1589.[92] Previously, he had paid a painter named Antonio thirteen lire six soldi to enliven the ornamental drapes in the entryway of Rini's house with "our coat of arms and medallions" and an additional eighteen lire to apply "chiaroscuro" decorations to five trunks and two curio cabinets.[93] Rini might not have been able to afford a painting by Bellini or a Titian, but he was a participant in Venice's visual culture and a mourner when that culture suffered erasures.

Disasters elicited Rini's commentary, but he also chronicled less fraught moments in the life of his city. Executions generally did not interest him, but Venice's relationship with the Ottomans did. Accordingly, he recorded the 1585 execution of the patrician galley captain Gabriel Emo, who had in the estimation of the Senate far exceeded his mandate in Algiers, "cutting to pieces many Turks, some of them women who belonged to the royal family of Algiers, and stealing their clothes, money, and jewels." With a sense of satisfaction in his city's legal process, Rini records that the "Most Excellent Council" passed sentence on Emo, who was then duly beheaded between the two columns in the piazzetta facing the lagoon.[94] Also in the category of civic events Rini included a brief report, written by his brother Scipione, of the 1585 Japanese embassy to Venice. In Scipione's estimation, these visitors were favorably impressed, at least with the hospitality of the city's confraternities. "The Japanese Indians," Scipione writes, "visited the Scuola della Carità, where the brethren of the Scuola Grande [di San Marco] gave them four decorated candles with candlesticks, a gift that they found delightful. And they said that they wanted to establish a similar confraternity in their own country."[95] Scipione's banal description supports almost uncannily Judith Brown's argument that Renaissance Italians, far from exoticizing the Japanese ambassadors, barely noticed them and showed little interest in exploring the cultural differences these visitors might have represented.[96] On the contrary, Brown points out that once we leave a few printed texts that did venture into exoticism and Orientalism more traditionally construed, Renaissance Italians envisioned a Japanese ambassador with "the heart of a European courtier and the soul of a Christian."[97] Consistently, then, Rini's journals offer in miniature form prevailing cultural currents.

Elections and deaths of doges also afforded opportunities for Rini to comment on civic affairs. While Rini did not editorialize at length, he made his views apparent. When Alvise Mocenigo became doge in 1571, Rini described the traditional ritual progress of the newly elected potentate throughout the piazza San Marco and his distribution of alms to the assembled crowd.[98] Adding his voice to what he characterized as the chorus of approval, Rini remarked that "everybody takes it as a given that he will be a truly glorious Doge, and maybe not less so than His Serenity Gritti of blessed memory. For three days straight, we were all celebrating in St. Mark's and running around the city. And the aforementioned Mocenigo is married to a woman from Ca' Marcello, so we have a Dogaressa, too."[99] Those optimistic predictions did not come to pass, owing to the onslaught of plague a few years later. Rini recorded the death of the doge himself shortly after the plague had abated in 1577, noting that Mocenigo received an honorable funerary oration by Lorenzo Massa (nephew of Nicolò Massa), by this point a secretary for the Senate.[100] Rini joined his fellow citizens in optimism at the election of Mocenigo's successor, Sebastian Valier, sharing the general hope that a new doge might mark the end of civic calamity. Rini deemed it auspicious that the forty-one voting officers of the conclave made their decision swiftly (within the space of twenty-four hours), choosing "the aforementioned Sebastian Venier, who was our naval captain in 1571 on that most solemn and memorable day when we were victorious against the Turks [the Battle of Lepanto]. And he had all 41 votes, something that is unheard of and united the whole city in surpassing joy."[101] Unfortunately, Venier lived only eight months past his election, dying in 1578, Rini observes, "after suffering for about eight days from a stroke. He was 82 years old. And, with the whole city in deep mourning at his passing, he was buried most honorably at Santa Maria degli Angeli on the island of Murano."[102] Although Rini seldom discussed the weather, on this occasion he followed good chronicle form in noting that on the day of Venier's funeral the rains were so torrential that the exequies had to be held at San Marco, making the climate a participant in the general mourning.[103]

For the most part, Rini's political commentary tended toward the positive. In the midst of economic and military disaster, to say nothing of epidemic disease, Rini still usually saw the doge as an embodiment of stability and the proper functioning of the civic order. When Rini did not care for a particular doge, however, he made that clear as well, aligning himself (as he did in the case of praise) with "everyone." Whereas Mocenigo, of whom Rini was an admirer, was not blamed for the plague, doges of whom Rini did not approve found themselves responsible for all the city's ills. Piero Loredan, who died in 1570 after a fire at the Arsenale, got a scorching farewell. "Everyone in Venice despised him," Rini remarked. "They say that he was the cause of the famine, death, and war that we have been suffering, as well as the fire at the Arsenal. He was buried at the church of San Iseppo."[104] In this case, Rini did not mention the funerary orator, nor did he give Loredan any honorifics. Stripping Loredan of "His Serenity," "Prencipe," "Clarissimo," and all the other titles naturally accorded to doges was the discursive equivalent of spitting on Loredan's grave.

Rini's experiment in poetry and his miniature chronicle of Venetian civic and cultural life serve, in the aggregate, as indications that even though he wrote such few words, he intended them for an audience beyond himself. Rini does exhibit many of the techniques that Pierre Hadot identifies as characteristic of philosophical autobiography, including interwoven composition, repetition of aphoristic expressions, idiosyncratic application of textual sources, remembrance of those who most influenced the writer's personal and ethical formation, and moral ruminations on individual political figures.[105] Yet our physician also departs from that paradigm in important ways. If we agree with Hadot that Marcus wrote exclusively for himself, or at most a transcendent Other, Rini seems to have had more literal audiences in mind as potential beneficiaries of his observations. His copying of sermons and his Stoic poem fit within the category of inner-directed model of self-writing that Hadot reconstructs; however, chronicling, recipe collecting, book purchases, and reportage of specific civic events turned Rini's attention to the sort of practical and historical material that a text such as Marcus's *Meditations* generally excludes.[106] All of which is to say that much more work can and should be done in considering the different models available to early-modern Europeans for writing about themselves.

Taking into account individual tastes and the limitations of his format, Rini accentuated many of the dimensions of cultural legitimacy that we have seen before: education, books, humanistic belonging, social ascent, the impulse to have one's say in a literary way. In and among quotidian transactions, we see him as a man of culture, often playing the role of reader or audience member, but occasionally trying his hand at some of the forms of writing he most admired and that formed such a large portion of his library: poetry, history, chronicles. However brief his memoranda, they were culturally significant, the things he wanted to remember owning, accomplishing, and noticing—and that he wished to be remembered for having owned, accomplished, noticed.

PER MEMORIA: A MONUMENT OF WORDS

The giornali of Alberto Rini defy any simple generic classification, as they encompass elements of ledgers, account books, *ricordanze,* diaries, and chronicles, even *zibaldoni* (miscellanies). These notebooks record moments in the history of a family and the history of a city; they attest to experiments in medical remedies and experiments in humanistic writing; they are records of other people's achievements; and they are self-writing. We see Rini paying rent, twice yearly, for the house that he and his brother leased from the nuns at the convent of San Zaccharia, and buying eggs, and tipping a cleaning woman who had given his regular maid a hand with "putting the house in order" before one hectic Christmas season—but we also see him tracking marriages inside and outside the family, buying books, and recording his experience of major events. The giornali are a discursive monument of Rini's life and times, however miniature that monument.

Rini's fusion of family history and business transactions is characteristic of Renaissance "account books," which as a genre can also indicate the encroachment of literary culture onto everyday affairs. Certainly, those who recorded their worlds had in mind an audience for those records, and often one beyond their immediate family. The recordkeeping fervor that inspired these booklets may have originated in the mercantile classes, but by the mid-fifteenth century, peasants, too, began to keep careful records of their important transactions and affairs. Duccio Balestracci, speaking of his central protagonist Benedetto del Massarizia, a Sienese peasant of the mid-fifteenth century who enlisted the aid of notaries to write his account books-cum-family memoirs, beautifully encapsulates the writing mania and fascination with the self that were characteristic of the Renaissance era. "He lived as so many others like him did," Balestracci writes, "but he also desired to keep some account of his life."[107] Alberto Rini shared Benedetto del Massarizia's desire to leave a record of his activities. This physician-chronicler also participated in the general spirit of artisan-merchants in fifteenth-century Italy who kept zibaldoni or "hodgepodge" books recording everything from gate tolls and exchange rates to recipes, devotions, and love lyrics, which Armando Petrucci sees as evidence of "a desire for extra-scholastic and autodidact acculturation that was both professional and ideological" and that he interprets as a craving on the part of ordinary men and women to inscribe "on a brief paper horizon of humble appearance the fundamental benchmarks of their culture and of their own presence in the society of the time."[108]

In Rini's own words, which he often repeated, he made his notes "per memoria," but it is clear that he meant them for more than his remembrance alone. Rini included information that would have been superfluous for himself or any close kin but that future readers would need. He was in no danger of forgetting that Scipione was his brother, for example, yet he always specifies the relationship. Nor would he have forgotten the fire in the ducal palace, or the paintings by Venetian masters that it had destroyed.

Some keepers of *ricordanze* exhibited this instinct to ensure their posterity through writing in a much more intense degree. Returning to Matthew Lundin's splendid analysis of Hermann Weinsberg's voluminous "memory books," we see a man who, working within this genre, pushed further into a form of writing that prefigured social history. Weinsberg hoped to leave to his heirs not only a record of what their own ancestors' lives had been like but also, for all future readers, an account of ordinary people—including his own urban middle ranks but also encompassing artisans, laborers, peasants—precisely the people that Weinsberg found frustratingly absent when he read histories and chronicles.[109]

Rini's commentary did not have that expansive aim, but he, too, recorded essential data for posterity, whether his own descendants or future chroniclers. As a reader and transcriber of chronicles himself, he knew the difficulties in finding the texture of daily life, or firsthand accounts of events to supplement the "facts" that state documents afford, and the generalizations that published histories furnish. Hence Rini's punctilious records of how many ballots each doge received, exactly how old they were, how long they stayed in office (down to the day), and, in most cases, the medical cause of their deaths, what "everybody" had thought about them, and who had enjoyed the honor of orating at their funerals. Hence also Rini's attempts, even within his space constraints, to record what the fire of 1577 destroyed, and to provide at least a sense of what it felt like to experience the conflagration.

And Rini chronicled himself. He did not indulge in lengthy interpretations of his life events, but he recorded his activities and significant transactions. Taken as a whole, these records form a self-portrait. What Rini does not say can be as revealing as what he does say. We do not learn about his medical fees or what advice he gave to his patients. Rini probably had separate account books for his professional work, as was standard at the time, but it is telling that nothing of his daily practice emerges in these miscellanies. Instead, Alberto Rini leaves us with the image of a reader, writer, and observer of his city.

Even through a medium even less conducive to literary expression than a testament, Rini found ways to highlight his intellectual and literary priorities. Particularly in the second journal, which covered the last twenty-five years of his life, Rini kept meticulous track of his book purchases, bibliographic loans, and interactions with the humanist Paolo Ramusio. In his second journal, Rini also remarked on civic events more consistently and expansively. Like Balestracci's Sienese peasant, Rini wanted to "keep some account of his life." But, even more like Lundin's eloquent lawyer, Rini had in mind an account not only of his economic and social transactions but also his participation in his city's cultural and literary ferment.

Alberto Rini's accounts thus provide us yet another vantage point onto early-modern cultural legitimacy. Massa took space in print and in his voluminous draft will to detail all the hassles and headaches he endured in building his family and proving his literary worth. Longo, in a far less agonistic vein, left in the more flexible format of his testaments cohesive relics of his accomplishments and philosophy. Rini, too, but in such few words, limned a miniature portrait of himself and his world.

In his memoranda, Rini gives us yet another answer to the question of what education did for early-modern Europeans, or at least for men and women in the middle ranks of Venice. Some of our protagonists found in education a means to prove the dignity of their professions, tighten their connections to the ennobling republic of letters, and sometimes help the family move forward socially as well. For others, above all Francesco Longo, education might have done all these things, but it also promised philosophical comfort. Education, as Longo represented it, was lived. Rini, in his turn, recalls these benefits while highlighting another. Our third physician shows us the peculiar confidence that an educated observer might feel even in distressing situations. Literary models and precedents offered the ability to derive larger meanings and connections, which meant that along with fear, subjects felt keen interest and a certain honor in noting the things—even the terrible things—they had seen and experienced. Observation and notation preserved one's existence and afforded a sense of participation in affairs both domestic and civic—or even global.

If Rini did not continue his family's lineage in the biological sense, he certainly did so in writing. Like Longo, Rini conceded that he was subject to the vicissitudes of fortune and divine will. Yet, like Longo and many others we have encountered, Rini found in the literary—in being educated, in accumulating humanistic books and precepts, in expressing what he thought in writing—a sense of sufficiency. Even in small acts of writing such as Rini performed, one proved educated merit in a tangible way. Like others who put pen to paper, or dictated to someone else who did, Alberto Rini had a reasonable hope that some trace of his cultural life would survive the dust and darkness of his tomb.

CONCLUSION

We have now seen many glimpses from the archival record of predominantly unheralded Venetians engaging with literary culture. Studying educational and bibliographic bequests, evidence of book ownership in household inventories and reading account books for cultural priorities have shown us avenues through which Venetians of the middling ranks sought and earned cultural legitimacy. Even if many questions remain about messer Francesco the retailer and manuscript borrower, we have seen that he was not alone in moving at once within mercantile and literary circles. By widening our documentary search, we approach Renaissance intellectual life without relying on a restricted roster of authors. The cultured people we have found in the archives turn us from humanistic production to wider patterns of literary consumption and, in the process, urge us to expand the boundaries we draw around Renaissance culture's spheres of influence. Far from construing commerce with literature as the preserve of scholars and writers, still less of the rich and noble, the testators and collectors we have met represented books and education as engines for their own social advancement and, in cases of less instrumental attitudes, a powerful confidence in personal and familial honor, as well as better hopes for remembrance in future generations.

The inherent rhetorical and philosophical rewards Venetians derived from their Renaissances may be more striking to intellectual historians and literary critics, but scholars at large may find the social power of literary endeavors an especially intriguing topic for future research.

Historians have long debated the boundaries of the possible for early-modern social mobility, which they have traditionally assessed by tabulating families' accumulation of wealth and their marriage strategies. Education gets short shrift in social history. We are regularly reminded that in medieval and early-modern Europe an ecclesiastical career brokered interactions with the higher echelons of society and that noncloistered "new men" in command of Latin also found advancement as secretaries to elites. In such cases, as David Herlihy has aptly summarized, skills "counted more than capital."[1] Yet the bulk of the analysis, even for Herlihy, rests on other forms of preferment: entrepreneurship, military service, and, above all, marital alliances.

In a similar vein, John Padgett has recently put debates about the permeability of the Florentine elite in the thirteenth and fourteenth centuries on a new footing through his analysis of tax censuses, city council records, genealogies, and other archival evidence relating to 1,697 families.[2] Padgett demonstrates impressive patterns of social advancement, in particular through families' accumulation of wealth, political offices, and (at intervals) their advantageous marriage alliances. Considering "upwardly mobile" marriages, Padgett emphasizes the decisive roles played by shared political faction and the lure of wealth. "Efforts to consolidate their own family positions," he explains, frequently "forced 'elites' . . . to reach down to marry middle-tier families, recruiting them as in-laws."[3] A closer analysis of those same middle-tier families might reveal that they won out not only because of their strengthening portfolios of financial and political capital but also because of their intellectual honor—proof of "nobility" in its own way, as contemporary discourse emphasized.

Marriage strategies also dominate the discussion of social mobility in the Venetian context. Dennis Romano has demonstrated a great deal of interconnection between the patrician and mercantile brackets of society. In particular, Romano sees in Venice a familiar European pattern of patrician men marrying wealthy nonpatrician women.[4] Following Romano, Alexander Cowan provides a rich account of Venetian social mobility, drawing on government documents in which patricians with doubtful pedigrees proved their nobility, or sub-patrician men and women proved that they fulfilled the requirements for marrying patricians, among the most important of these proofs being evidence that the family had not performed manual labor for at least three generations.[5] Cowan demonstrates a regular current of interclass alliances. He also adds to the usual factors for social advancement a quality he terms "manners," meaning a fusion of moral and social respectability that education (in the sense of upbringing) conferred on its recipients, making them viable potential mates for their superiors. Ultimately, however, the essential forces driving this mobility remain the accumulation of wealth and advantageous marriage alliances.

Cash, real estate, land, and marriage strategies no doubt played essential roles in the social transactions of early-modern Venice, but so did Renaissance culture's more abstract conceptions of merit and worth, topics generally reserved for intellectual historians and literary critics. We have learned here, however, that the metaphorical nobility conferred by interaction with education, books, and ideas was not just a pipe dream in the republic of letters but instead had tangible power. Men and women of the upwardly mobile artisanal and mercantile classes voiced the notion that education held a central place in the portfolio of assets that could speed their kin to better things. Venetians used the phrase *uomo da bene* to articulate the social power of the literary, bridging general virtues such as honesty with academic or literary attainments. In context of questions about citizenship and legitimacy, the Paduan pharmacists who called Francesco Longo's father a *uomo da bene* indicated that Pietro Longo dealt honestly in business and had no scandal attached to him—we hear echoes of Cowan's conception of manners here—but they also spoke of his having more remarkable achievements. We have also seen this phrase attached to discussions of the liberal arts by parents stating that an advanced education would help a son become a *uomo da bene*. The phrase evoked a mutually reinforcing relationship between social and intellectual respectability. The humanities, in short, proved a person's cultural legitimacy. And that cultural legitimacy might, in some cases, compensate for social demerits such as an artisanal background or biological illegitimacy, as well as dignify occupations or professions tainted by their association with mercenary gain or the marketplace—associations that still troubled medicine.

We have conceived of literature in the Renaissance as primarily ornamental for those who were not card-carrying members of the humanist elite.[6] The physicians, priests, merchants, and artisans we have met through the archives urge rethinking that conceptualization. Renaissance ideals and concepts were prized and practiced in concrete terms, as a means of enhancing a family's honor and, in due course, its social standing. Francesco Longo experienced that narrative, though he does not say so. Massa, Superchio, and Rini provided details. Like Superchio, Massa improved on his mercantile origins, managing though his medical practice and his prolific publications to get one nephew married to a noblewoman, another into a legal career, and even his illegitimate daughter married into a patrician family with considerable landholdings. His detailed instructions regarding the education of his grandson tell us that he was determined to see these improvements continue, through Maria, along what he termed his *linea retta*. Massa was atypical in tracing his biological line through his daughter, but very much with the times in emphasizing cultural no less than financial or marital strategies for family advancement. The apothecary Pietro Longo shared Massa's strategy, ensuring that his son would attend university. We have met other families of higher artisans, merchants, and unremarkable *cittadini* with similar stories. We have seen men of citizen rank pushing their children into lateral achievement as physicians, or marginal advancement as lawyers. But we have also seen cases of dramatic movement, such as daughters of physicians marrying landed nobility or illegitimate daughters marrying citizens. Educated men and women could change roles even within the ostensibly rigid hierarchy of Venice and against formidable obstacles, the taint of manual labor or rough commerce in one's ancestry, or illegitimacy. Armed with the collateral of an engraved silver basin, the servant of a secondhand goods dealer could even borrow Greek manuscripts from the collection at San Marco.

In Renaissance Venice, cultural legitimacy could be worth as much as money, land, or even blood in the calculation of honor. Let us return to one case, the Peranda family, as a last look at the social power of books and education. In 1585, the physician Giovan Battista Peranda dictated a will in which he made many bequests to friends and colleagues, but his most remarkable legacy went to his protégée and informal adoptee: "I leave to Giovan Battista, son of Pietro, my valet, and Marietta, our longtime maid, if he studies (as I hope he will do) all of my books and everything else in my study."[7] Peranda's wife and executor, Laura Foscarini, underscored her husband's intentions in her own will of 1587. Foscarini clarified that the junior Giovan Battista should be understood as her adopted son.[8] This patrician daughter and physician's wife also stressed that academic attainment would move the young man forward socially, even more than her considerable wealth and influence. While not as doctrinaire as the physician Valerio Superchio, or even the priest Paulo Pincio, Foscarini nonetheless leaves no doubt that Giovan Battista's future depended on his accumulation of cultural legitimacy. She not only made her adopted son her universal heir; she earmarked hundreds of ducats for her executors to spend in the years until he reached his majority on his clothing, school expenses, and, "when the time comes, the cost of sending him to the *Studium* [Padua] and seeing to it that he studies law." Legal studies once again appear in a medical family's strategies for moving the next generation into a higher echelon of the civil professions. In concluding, she beseeches her executors to "take care above all else that Giovan Battista study, so that he may be called 'His Excellency' and become a man of good reputation and honored [*homo da bene et honorato*]."[9] Learning and university credentials again emerge as the linchpins in a family strategy for ensuring that a promising adolescent laboring under a social defect might earn credibility as a "man of the right sort."

Signora Foscarini Peranda had absolute faith in the honor that Giovan Battista's studies would confer on him. That faith may well have come from reading humanistic material, but it also came from experience. Her husband had been a physician of good repute, but he was not a patrician; her family, the Foscarini, was not merely patrician but ducal. Termed "magnifica" even by her husband, this testator played the ingénue in one story of educational social mobility and the matriarch in another. She put her cash, property, and social networks in the hands of a promising young man who by parentage belonged to the ranks of laborers and servants but who had impressed her husband. Still, realizing that adopting Giovan Battista and lavishing money and property on him would be less important than a university degree for his accumulation of merit and status, Signora Peranda emphasized that, given his origins, he must have a doctorate to earn sufficient merit for becoming "His Excellency, a man of good reputation and honored."

Giovan Battista Peranda fulfilled most of his adoptive mother's hopes. He did earn his doctorate and enjoyed a good reputation, even if, in the end, he did not study law. Instead, the young man chose to follow his adoptive father and namesake, graduating from the Paduan *Studium* in 1602 with a doctorate in arts and medicine.[10] By the late 1630s, Peranda was serving as counsel to Venice's College of Surgeons, as we learn from several witchcraft trials in which witnesses mentioned having sought his medical advice when dealing with potentially "supernatural illnesses."[11] Considering that he began life as the son of a carpenter and a maid, the degree of trust and authority that the junior Giovan Battista Peranda's career involved offers striking exemplification of the cultural, social, and professional credibility that came with a university degree.

Stories like Peranda's reinforce the critical importance of intellectual achievement in Renaissance calculations of merit. Yet I hope that *Everyday Renaissances* may serve not only as an impetus to include considerations of education in social history but also as a model for analyzing social constraints, nuances of temperament, and objectives in the accumulation and uses of honor. Beyond their instrumental applications, humanistic ideals brought a discursive conception of posterity. Petrarch's autobiographical letter to posterity offered one influential model.[12] We have seen a similar spirit for creating textual monuments in the wills of our own protagonists. The transmission of property to bodily heirs remained important. And, for those who had the means, elaborate funerals and monuments of marble and brass also promised to remind future generations of personal and familial achievements. Yet with humanism came what we might term a Petrarchan, or indeed in the first instance Ciceronian, conception of the written word as a means of ensuring remembrance. In one of Cicero's later letters, a crucial source of inspiration for Petrarch, the old orator and statesman fretted about his posthumous reputation, begging the historian Lucius Lucceius to include him in the account of the civil wars that Lucius was just then finishing. Despite the many other "monuments" he left, Cicero understood his best hope for commemoration would be the written word. If this historian could not accommodate the request, Cicero feared that his only alternative would be to write his own life story, which (he said) he was loath to do.[13]

The individuals we have encountered here conducted their own anxious conversations with posterity through the medium of paper. Cicero and his brilliant early-modern descendants could call on either their own resources or else contemporary historians to commemorate their achievements in print. But less illustrious and less erudite men and women found ways to do the same. Thanks to Matthew Lundin, we now understand Hermann Weinsberg's seven thousand pages of personal, family, and civic history as an appropriation of just such a Ciceronian conception of posterity, as filtered through contemporary humanist writing.[14] Our Venetian subjects similarly wrote memorials of themselves and their families—far shorter accounts, in most cases, but effective and, for the modern historian, perhaps even more compelling on account of their humble brevity. Our subjects shared with someone like Weinsberg—or, for that matter, people like Cicero and Petrarch—the notion that, beyond their bodily heirs, their posterity lay in their words, whether lengthy original compositions or just a book inventory, a testament, a note in a ledger. Family documents might seem fragile materials for such important matters. Petrarch, after all, had chosen the ostensibly more durable method of circulating an elegant Latin epistle to set his own record straight. Yet inventories, testaments, and even account books promised to endure. Tethered at once to family and state, as well as to real property, legal machinery, and Christian conceptions of the afterlife, these materials became monuments, in their own way, more lasting than bronze.

Of all the fragments of Renaissance culture we have found in Venetian households, those of physicians have taught us most about commitments to humanistic conceptions of legitimacy and posterity. In their eloquent last wills and testaments, the self-made man of letters Nicolò Massa and the philosophical Francesco Longo counseled and informed future generations. Their families would have heard the lessons in person, probably many times. Like Rini's giornali, then, these documents were not addressed just to kin but also to whatever audience we envision when we account for our lives.[15] In these acts of self-writing, the speakers move from the mundane to focus on the mind, at least as concerned with the preservation of their books and precepts as with their other possessions. Humanistic aspiration changed the nature of these texts. What might have been quotidian records of property and expenditure became Renaissances, writ small.

Where might scholars take this book's method of tracing Renaissances writ small in diverse archival materials, as well as its framing concepts of testamentary humanism and cultural legitimacy? As we work toward an even clearer understanding of the literary lives of those who were not among their era's celebrities, we would do well to interweave testaments, inventories, and account books into our analyses. Much excellent work has been done on the material Renaissance. I would urge us to keep looking for books alongside clothing, furnishings, works of art, and the other consumer goods that tend to predominate in studies of material culture. In work that explicitly considers the materiality of books, such as William Sherman's exposition of marginalia, we must also take care to keep broader patterns of both book ownership and literary expression in view.[16] Sherman, for instance, illuminates the reading practices of Elizabethan England by tracking manicules and other signs that readers used to mark the passages they found most significant in a wide range of texts. Yet in many cases we cannot know who those particular readers were (even if he divines their general status from penmanship and other indications), nor does Sherman delve much into the frequency with which such texts appeared in book inventories. Similarly, Jeffrey Todd Knight has diversified our image of early-modern book culture and collecting practices by innovative interpretation of the texts' many packaging options.[17] The defect connected to the merits of studies rooted in material analysis are that questions concerning what owners and readers might have done with their books and the knowledge they found in them play a secondary role. Reading testaments and other family documents for the literary keeps these other questions in view.

If my exploration of cultural legitimacy has focused on the sixteenth century, this is by no means to suggest that this era was uniquely propitious. While I do contend that the centrality of humanistic tenets obtaining by the late Renaissance played an important role in shaping contemporary definitions of merit and legitimacy, similar fusions of intellectual, literary, and social ideals operated long before Petrarch and long after Galileo. Indeed, cultural legitimacy might also prove more useful a heuristic tool for ancient and medieval protagonists than concepts such as Bourdieu's "cultural capital," which rely analogically if not functionally on an economic system that did not exist in those contexts any more than they did in Renaissance Italy.

Nor was the search for cultural legitimacy geographically bounded. Every locality has its peculiarities, but the general contours of intellectual and literary life even in a city as particular as Venice map onto many urban centers in the early-modern world. As we have seen, comparison between my findings and those of Albert Labarre, Renata Ago, and Lorna Weatherill, among others, suggests similar topographies of book owners in France, in other parts of Italy, and in Britain. Comparison between some of my own subjects and Matthew Lundin's fascinating Cologne lawyer has underscored the potentially transregional nature of cultural legitimacy as an idea, bibliomania and graphomania as practices, and anxious rhetoric of honor as the standard expressive register of those who had educations but little else to distinguish them. So, too, Dana Sajdi has found among Ottoman "nouveau literates" much the same correlation between rise in academic status and social mobility.[18]

As work continues, university towns might prove richer sites than urban centers for finding aspirants to cultural legitimacy. Beyond the higher volume of records generated by students and scholars, town members might well have attended to and perhaps even kept pace with local standards of merit shaped by conceptions of intellectual honor. As fascinated as I am by the libraries of Massa, Quattrocchi, or Rini, no less than the far more diminutive collections of an artisan's wife such as Catharina, widow of the goldsmith Castelino, I must concede that, in terms of numbers, even the largest Venetian libraries pale in comparison to those we find at Padua. To take only one example, we have the stunning collection of books, art, and antiquities compiled by Pietro Bembo and interpreted by Paula Findlen.[19] Perhaps tellingly, Bembo chose to maintain that collection in Padua, despite the fact that his primary residence was in Venice and by the latter part of his career he lived in Rome. Bembo may have wanted to keep his cultural investments where they signified the most, spatially linked to one of Europe's premier universities.

The concepts of testamentary humanism and cultural legitimacy might also prove useful as work continues on the transmission of art, as well as music, among people who were not their era's most remarkable collectors. Art historians have recently shown that while the ranks of book owners (at least those revealed in inventories) hover around 20 percent of any given sample, those same inventories reveal that nearly every household had at least one artifact of visual culture.[20] Art objects, and for that matter musical ones, might also be read as forms of cultural legitimacy, or signs of people seeking it. Following Renata Ago and others, interdisciplinary analysis of books, art, music, and household furnishings will no doubt yield an even sharper image of the cultural lives of early-modern men and women. But we must continue to ask questions of the sort that have driven my own study, not only looking for ownership but also examining the uses to which owners put their treasures. In particular, we should keep familial, occupational, and economic pressures a part of our analytical frameworks. We must ask for what ends or audiences an individual might have invested in a print landscape, just as we have asked what an innkeeper wanted with the *Divine Comedy,* or what a secondhand goods dealer hoped to do with manuscripts of Greek philosophy.[21] Although individual taste, aesthetics, pleasure, and innate desire for edification no doubt informed these acquisitions, nonetheless if we want our hermeneutic tools to measure the human in the humanistic as completely as possible, they must accommodate consideration of the pressures to earn honor, belong to a respected intellectual lineage, enjoy advancement. These pressures affected not only those positioned in or near the governing elite of the republic of letters but also those inhabiting its peripheries.

Above all, I hope that this study will encourage early modernists to think anew about connections between books and honor across cities and regions. We will not always unearth proof that reading publics found (or did not find) the pleasure, edification, or social mobility they sought. This is another reason that cultural capital as a conceptual tool proves too limiting: Much of its utility lies in processes of conversion, making success or failure integral to the argument. By contrast, my own emphasis on a wider conception of legitimacy and lineage, on degrees of belonging, has greater flexibility, accommodating the relative paucities of evidentiary material for the early-modern period and especially for those outside the ranks of the robustly enfranchised. In itself, possessing education or books offered proof of merit, of belonging to circles of "the right sort." In some cases, the educated and the owners of books go on to tell us, or other documents help us see, the ways in which those possessions preserved or bettered their own lives and the prospects for their kin. Innkeepers, wives of perfumers, pharmacists, secondhand goods dealers, parish priests, physicians—Venetians from all these categories believed and invested in cultural legitimacy. Those far from the ranks of the enfranchised shared with the privileged a confidence in education's ennobling powers. That shared confidence expresses with a new force and clarity the reach of humanistic ideals in late Renaissance Venice. As research continues, I suspect that we will keep finding that same confidence in localities far beyond La Serenissima and, indeed, far beyond Europe.

ABBREVIATIONS

AAUP	Archivio Antico dell'Università, Padua
ASP	Archivio Storico Patriarcale, Venice
ASV	Archivio di Stato, Venice
BNM	Biblioteca Nazionale di San Marco (Marciana), Venice
CI	Cancelleria Inferiore, Miscellanea Notai Diversi, Inventari (ASV)
DER	Derelitti (IRE)
GP	Giudici di Petizion, Inventari (ASV)
IRE	Archivio IRE (Istituzioni di Ricovero e di Educazione), Venice
NT	Notarile Testamenti (ASV)
ZIT	Zitelle (IRE)

NOTE ON THE SOURCES

All translations from the Italian and Latin are my own, unless otherwise indicated. I have retained the spellings, diacritics, and punctuation of the original sources quoted in the notes, except when the meaning would have been obscured without alteration. I have, however, used modern phrasing and punctuation in the translations. Original language quotations from archival sources and rare print publications appear in the notes. In the interest of space, however, I have not provided original language quotations from texts that are relatively accessible.

NOTES

INTRODUCTION

1. Jacob Burckhardt, *The Civilization of the Renaissance in Italy,* trans. C. G. C. Middlemore (New York: Dover Publications, 2010), esp. 217–222 and 240–243.
2. The classic study of the phenomenon is Lauro Martines, *Power and Imagination: City States in Renaissance Italy* (Baltimore, MD: Johns Hopkins University Press, 1988). For an alternative viewpoint, emphasizing artistic and literary agency, see Diana Robin, *Filelfo in Milan, Writings 1451–1477* (Princeton, NJ: Princeton University Press, 1991).
3. This line of questioning emerges with particular clarity in considerations of women's education; see especially Lisa Jardine, "Women Humanists: Education for What?," in *From Humanism to the Humanities: Education and the Liberal Arts in Fifteenth- and Sixteenth-Century Europe,* ed. Anthony Grafton and Lisa Jardine (London: Duckworth, 1986), 29–57.
4. BNM, "prestiti di Manoscritti Marciani," Cod. Lat. XIV.23 (=4660), fol.15r: "Messer Francesco de Polo tien bottega di strazaria apresso Therologio a S. Marco ha havuto [. . .] il libro greco in pergameno ditto Proculo Platonico in la Theologia de Platon et Il comento de Jerocleo sopra li aurei versi di Pythagora, portoli Zuane da V.a suo fante in ditta botega che l'have da mi, et Io per segnal ho havuto uno bacile de rasini dargento."
5. My conception of "cultural legitimacy" naturally differs from definitions in modern public policy and business, where the phrase indicates a branding strategy in a specific market context or a state program for gaining the trust of indigenous peoples. In the one sense, see, for instance, the Hartman Group's 2004 pamphlet on "Cultural Legitimacy" (http://www.hartman-group.com/publications/white-papers/cultural-legitimacy) or Surrey International

Law Centre's 2011 conference, "Cultural Legitimacy and the International Law and Policy on Climate Change" (http://www.ias.surrey.ac.uk/workshops/silc/); in the other, "Building and Maintaining Cultural Legitimacy," in the Reconciliation Australia Governance Toolkit (http://www.reconciliation.org.au/governance/resource/building-and-maintaining-cultural-legitimacy). See below for a further distinction between my usage of *legitimacy* and its common use in political discourse.

6. See especially Jutta Sperling, *Convents and the Body Politic in Late Renaissance Venice* (Chicago: University of Chicago Press, 2000); Stanley Chojnacki, "Marriage Regulation in Venice, 1420–1535" and "Subaltern Patriarchs: Patrician Bachelors," in *Women and Men in Renaissance Venice: Twelve Essays on Patrician Society,* ed. Stanley Chojnacki (Baltimore, MD: Johns Hopkins University Press, 2000), 53–75 and 244–256. For a broader view, see Luciano Pezzolo, "The Venetian Economy, 1400–1797," in *A Companion to Venetian History, 1400–1797,* ed. Eric Dursteler (Leiden: Brill, 2013), 255–290.
7. On print culture in Italy, see Brian Richardson, *Printing, Writers and Readers in Renaissance Italy* (Cambridge: Cambridge University Press, 1999), esp. 137–142; Marino Zorzi, "La circolazione del libro a Venezia nel Cinquecento: biblioteche private e pubbliche," *Ateneo veneto* 177 (1990): 117–189 (for the range of figures cited here, see 165); Marino Zorzi, "Le biblioteche veneziane, espressione di una singolare civiltà," in *The Books of Venice/Il libro veneziano,* ed. Lisa Pon and Craig Kallendorf (Venice: Biblioteca Nazionale Marciana and Oak Knoll Press, 2007), 1–30; Andrew Pettegree, *The Book in the Renaissance* (New Haven, CT: Yale University Press, 2012), 60–62, 66–67, and 254–255.
8. Christopher Celenza, "Poliziano's *Lamia* in Context," in *Angelo Poliziano's* Lamia: *Text, Translation and Introductory Studies* (Leiden: Brill, 2010), 45.
9. Ramusio also consulted manuscripts at San Marco that were all available in print. See BNM, Cod. Lat. XIV.22 (=4482), fols. 3v and 15v.
10. A defining feature of Bourdieu's thought throughout his career, "cultural capital" receives the most extensive explication and substantiation in *La Distinction: Critique social du jugement* (1979) which I have consulted in Richard Nice's translation, *Distinction: A Social Critique of the Judgement of Taste* (Cambridge, MA: Harvard University Press, 1984). See also Bourdieu's *The Field of Cultural Production: Essays on Art and Literature,* ed. Randal Johnson (New York: Polity Press, 1993), esp. 7, 43–54, 170–195, and 270n24.
11. Bourdieu, *Distinction,* 125–168 and 291; Bourdieu, *Field,* 161–175.
12. On dissatisfaction with Bourdieu's economic emphasis (if not determinism), see David Swartz, *Culture and Power: The Sociology of Pierre Bourdieu* (Chicago: University of Chicago Press, 1997), 78–82.
13. Renata Ago, *Il gusto delle cose. Una storia degli oggetti nella Roma del Seicento* (Rome: Donzelli Editore, 2006).
14. Lorna Weatherill, "The Meaning of Consumer Behaviour in Late Seventeenth- and Early Eighteenth-Century England," in *Consumption and the World of Goods* (London: Routledge, 1993), 206–227.

15. Ago, *Il gusto delle cose,* 75, 187, 220, and 214.
16. Ibid., 187.
17. Bourdieu, *Distinction,* 11–96; quotation at 69.
18. For developing definitions and applications of this concept, see especially ibid., 101–115, 123, and 172–173; Bourdieu, *Field,* 6–7, 61–72, and 181–191; for synthetic treatment, see Swartz, *Culture and Power,* 35, 100–103, and 197.
19. For the plight of the autodidact in Bourdieu's schema, see *Distinction,* 84–85 and 328–331.
20. Ago, *Il gusto delle cose,* 214.
21. Ibid., 219.
22. For determinism in Bourdieu's conception of the social *agon,* see Swartz, *Culture and Power,* 75–82.
23. An excellent recent study of the problem is Laurence Fontaine, *The Moral Economy: Poverty, Credit and Trust in Early Modern Europe* (Cambridge: Cambridge University Press, 2014). See also Mario Biagioli, *Galileo's Instruments of Credit: Telescopes, Images, Secrecy* (Chicago: University of Chicago Press, 2007); Steven Shapin, *A Social History of Truth: Civility and Science in Seventeenth-Century England* (Chicago: University of Chicago Press, 1995); Dale Kent, *Friendship, Love and Trust in Renaissance Florence* (Cambridge, MA: Harvard University Press, 2009).
24. On humanist uses of Plutarch in seeking advancement, see Elizabeth McCahill, *Reviving the Eternal City: Rome and the Paper Court, 1420–1447* (Cambridge, MA: Harvard University Press, 2013), 51–55 and 176; as well as Elizabeth McCahill, "Finding a Job as a Humanist: The Epistolary Collection of Lapo da Castiglionchio the Younger," *Renaissance Quarterly* 57, no. 4 (2004): 1314–1316. See also Christopher Celenza, "Parallel Lives: Plutarch's *Lives,* Lapo da Castiglionchio the Younger (1405–1438) and the Art of Italian Renaissance Translation," *Illinois Classical Studies* 22 (1997): 121–155; Vito Giustiniani, "Sulle Traduzioni Latine delle 'Vite' di Plutarco nel Quattrocento," *Rinascimento* 1 (1961): 3–62; Marianne Pade, "Sulla Fortuna delle Vite di Plutarco nell'Umanesimo Italiano del Quattrocento," *Fontes* 1 (1998): 101–116; as well as Pade's magisterial two-volume treatment of the topic, *The Reception of Plutarch's Lives in Fifteenth-Century Italy* (Copenhagen: Museum Tusculanum Press, University of Copenhagen, 2007).
25. Nancy Siraisi, *History, Medicine and the Traditions of Renaissance Learning* (Ann Arbor: University of Michigan Press, 2007); Nancy Siraisi, *Communities of Learned Experience* (Baltimore, MD: Johns Hopkins University Press, 2013). See also her own acknowledged model, T. C. Price Zimmerman, *Paolo Giovio: The Historian and the Crisis of the Sixteenth Century* (Princeton, NJ: Princeton University Press, 1995).
26. This is particularly true in Douglas Biow, *Doctors, Ambassadors, Secretaries: Humanism and the Professions in Renaissance Italy* (Chicago: University of Chicago Press, 2002).
27. Bourdieu, *Distinction,* 84.

28. Paul Grendler, "The Italian Renaissance in the Past Seventy Years: Humanism, Social History and the Early Modern in Anglo-American and Italian Scholarship," in *The Italian Renaissance in the Twentieth Century: Acts of an International Conference, Florence, Villa I Tatti, June 9–11 1999,* ed. Allen J. Grieco et al. (Florence: Leo S. Olschki, 2002), 3–23.
29. Peter Gay, "The Social History of Ideas: Ernst Cassirer and After," in *The Critical Spirit: Essays in Honor of Herbert Marcuse,* ed. Herbert Marcuse, Kurt H. Wolff, and Barrington Moore (Boston: Beacon Press, 1967), 106–120.
30. Roger Chartier, *The Order of Books: Readers, Authors and Libraries in Europe between the Fourteenth and Eighteenth Centuries,* trans. Lydia G. Cochrane (Stanford, CA: Stanford University Press, 1992); Peter Burke, *A Social History of Knowledge: From Gutenberg to Diderot* (Malden, MA: Polity Press, 2000); Peter Burke, *Languages and Communities in Early Modern Europe* (Cambridge: Cambridge University Press, 2004).
31. Marco Biagioli, *Galileo Courtier: The Practice of Science in the Culture of Absolutism* (Chicago: University of Chicago Press, 1994); Biagioli, *Galileo's Instruments of Credit.*
32. Shapin, *Social History of Truth.*
33. Paula Findlen, *Possessing Nature: Museums, Collecting and Scientific Culture in Early Modern Italy* (Berkeley: University of California Press, 1996).
34. Lauro Martines, *Power and Imagination: The Social World of the Florentine Humanists, 1390–1460* (Toronto: University of Toronto Press, 2011); Lauro Martines, *Strong Words: Writing and Social Strain in the Italian Renaissance* (Baltimore, MD: Johns Hopkins University Press, 2003); Robin, *Filelfo in Milan;* Christopher Celenza, *The Lost Renaissance: Humanists, Historians and Latin's Legacy* (Baltimore, MD: Johns Hopkins University Press, 2005), chap. 3; Brian Maxson, *The Humanist World of Renaissance Florence* (Cambridge: Cambridge University Press, 2014).
35. Diana Robin, *Publishing Women: Salons, the Presses and the Counter-Reformation in Sixteenth-Century Italy* (Chicago: University of Chicago Press, 2007); Julie Campbell, *Literary Circles and Gender in Early Modern Europe: A Cross-Cultural Approach* (Aldershot, UK: Ashgate, 2006); Sarah Gwyneth Ross, *The Birth of Feminism: Woman as Intellect in Renaissance Italy and England* (Cambridge, MA: Harvard University Press, 2009); Carol Pal, *Republic of Women: Rethinking the Republic of Letters in the Seventeenth Century* (Cambridge: Cambridge University Press, 2012).
36. Albert Labarre, *Le livre dans la vie amiénoise du seizième siècle: L'enseignement des inventaires après décès (1503–1576)* (Paris: Nauwelaerts, 1971).
37. Robert Darnton, "In Search of Enlightenment: Recent Attempts to Create a Social History of Ideas," *Journal of Modern History* 43, no. 1 (1971): 113–132.
38. Among many contributions, see Robert Darnton, *The Great Cat Massacre and Other Episodes in French Cultural History* (New York: Basic Books, 1984); Robert Darnton, *The Forbidden Bestsellers of Prerevolutionary France* (New York: Norton, 1996).

39. Robert Darnton, "A Police Inspector Sorts His Files: The Anatomy of the Republic of Letters," in *The Great Cat Massacre and Other Episodes in French Cultural History* (New York: Basic Books, 1984), 145–190.
40. Ibid., 154.
41. Ibid., 150 and 152.
42. Darnton, "Readers Respond to Rousseau," in *The Great Cat Massacre and Other Episodes in French Cultural History* (New York: Basic Books, 1984), 215–251.
43. Darnton, *The Great Cat Massacre,* 258.
44. Chartier, *Order of Books,* 7.
45. Ibid., 8; in the original version, *L'ordre des livres: Lecteurs, auteurs, bibliothèques en Europe entre xive et xviiie siècle* (Aix-en-Provence, France: Alinea, 1992), 19 (hereafter *L'ordre*).
46. Chartier, *Order of Books,* 8; *L'ordre,* 19.
47. Ibid.
48. Chartier's translator has given *maniés* a positive rendering, but while it can mean "manipulated" a more common English translation would be "handled." The term invokes manual culture and gives the locution a condescending valence.
49. Ibid., 19. Chartier's paradigmatic author is Diderot. His paradigmatic "library without walls" the multivolume *Bibliotheca universalis,* a compendium of all works known as of the late sixteenth century in Latin, Greek, and Hebrew, compiled by the botanist-humanist Conrad von Gesner.
50. Peter Burke, *Popular Culture in Early Modern Europe,* rev. ed. (Aldershot, UK: Ashgate, 2009).
51. Peter Burke, *The Historical Anthropology of Early Modern Italy: Essays on Perception and Communication* (Cambridge: Cambridge University Press, 1987), esp. 113.
52. See especially Armando Petrucci, *Writers and Readers in Medieval Italy: Studies in the History of Written Culture,* trans. Charles M. Radding (New Haven, CT: Yale University Press, 1995).
53. Weatherill, "Meaning of Consumer Behaviour," 207.
54. Burke, *Social History of Knowledge,* 2.
55. Ibid., 14.
56. Ibid.
57. Ibid., 181–192.
58. Lisa Jardine, *Worldly Goods: A New History of the Renaissance* (New York: W. W. Norton, 1998); Evelyn Welch, *Shopping in the Renaissance: Consumer Cultures in Italy, 1400–1600* (New Haven, CT: Yale University Press, 2009).
59. Weatherill, "Meaning of Consumer Behaviour," 206–227.
60. Pamela Smith, *The Body of the Artisan: Art and Experience in the Scientific Revolution* (Chicago: University of Chicago Press, 2006); Pamela Long, *Artisan/Practitioners and the Rise of the New Sciences, 1400–1600* (Corvallis: Oregon State University Press, 2011). See also Pamela Smith and Paula Findlen, eds., *Merchants and Marvels: Commerce, Science and Art in Early Modern Europe* (London: Routledge, 2002).

61. For good synthetic assessment, see Pettegree, *Book in the Renaissance.*
62. Ann Blair, *Too Much to Know: Managing Scholarly Information before the Modern Age* (New Haven, CT: Yale University Press, 2010).
63. William H. Sherman, *Used Books: Marking Readers in Renaissance England* (Philadelphia: University of Pennsylvania Press, 2007). In a similar vein, Jeffrey Todd Knight looks at the myriad packaging possibilities for early-modern books to make claims about readers' different approaches to literary material; see his *Bound to Read: Compilations, Collections and the Making of Renaissance Literature* (Philadelphia: University of Pennsylvania Press, 2013).
64. Pettegree, *Book in the Renaissance.*
65. Petrucci, *Writers and Readers,* 222–223. Here Petrucci draws on Christian Bec, *Les marchands écrivains. Affaires et humanisme à Florence, 1375–1434* (Paris: Mouton, 1967), 394–415.
66. Christian Bec, *Les livres des Florentines (1413–1608)* (Florence: Leo S. Olschki, 1984). See also Bec, *Les marchands écrivains.*
67. Ago, *Il gusto delle cose.*
68. Isabella Cecchini, "Collezionismo e mondo materiale," *Il collezionismo d'arte a Venezia* 2 (2008): 165–191; on books, apart from their numerical tabulation, see 178.
69. Susan Connell, "Books and Their Owners in Venice, 1345–1480," *Journal of the Warburg and Courtauld Institutes* 35 (1972): 163–186; Marino Zorzi, "La circolazione del libro a Venezia nel Cinquecento: biblioteche private e pubbliche," *Ateneo veneto* 177 (1990): 117–189.
70. Jonathan Rose, *The Intellectual Life of the British Working Classes,* 2nd ed. (New Haven, CT: Yale University Press, 2010), xi.
71. Carlo Ginzburg, *The Cheese and the Worms: The Cosmos of a Sixteenth-Century Miller,* trans. John and Anne Tedeschi (Baltimore, MD: Johns Hopkins University Press, 1980).
72. Duccio Balestracci, *Renaissance in the Fields: Family Memoirs of a Fifteenth-Century Tuscan Peasant,* trans. Paolo Squatriti and Betsy Merideth (University Park: Pennsylvania State University Press, 1999).
73. Celenza, *Lost Italian Renaissance,* 69 and 79.
74. David Ruderman, "Between High and Low Cultures: Echoes of the New Science in the Writings of Judah Del Bene and Azariah Figo," in *Jewish Thought and Scientific Discovery in Early Modern Europe* (New Haven, CT: Yale University Press, 1995); Siraisi, *History, Medicine and the Traditions of Renaissance Learning,* especially the discussion of Hartman Schedel's redaction of the Nuremberg Chronicle, 19.
75. See especially Paul Oskar Kristeller, "Humanism and Scholasticism in the Italian Renaissance," *Byzantion* 24 (1947): 346–374; Ronald Witt, *In the Footsteps of the Ancients: The Origins of Humanism from Lovato to Bruni* (Leiden: Brill, 2000); Ronald Witt, *The Two Latin Cultures and the Foundation of Renaissance Humanism in Medieval Italy* (Cambridge: Cambridge University Press, 2012).
76. Anthony Grafton and Lisa Jardine, eds., *From Humanism to the Humanities: The Institutionalizing of the Liberal Arts in Fifteenth- and Sixteenth-Century Europe*

(Cambridge, MA: Harvard University Press, 1987); Anthony Grafton and Ann Blair, *The Transmission of Culture in Early Modern Europe* (Philadelphia: University of Pennsylvania Press, 1990); Anthony Grafton, *Commerce with the Classics: Ancient Books and Renaissance Readers* (Ann Arbor: University of Michigan Press, 1997); Craig Kallendorf, *Virgil and the Myth of Venice: Books and Readers in the Italian Renaissance* (Oxford: Clarendon Press, 1999); Jill Kraye, ed., *The Cambridge Companion to Renaissance Humanism* (Cambridge: Cambridge University Press, 2007), xv; Adam Shear, "Judah Moscato's Scholarly Self-Image," in *Cultural Intermediaries: Jewish Intellectuals in Early Modern Italy,* ed. David Ruderman and Giuseppe Veltri (Philadelphia: University of Pennsylvania Press, 2004), 157–160.

77. James Hankins, "Humanism in the Vernacular: The Case of Leonardo Bruni," in *Humanism and Creativity in the Renaissance,* ed. Christopher Celenza and Kenneth Gouwens (Leiden: Brill, 2006), 11–29. See also Hankins's analysis of Plato's fortuna among a wide range of scholars and readers in his magisterial *Plato in the Italian Renaissance* (Leiden: Brill Academic Publishing, 1990), 95–97 and 363, and his "Lorenzo de' Medici's *De summo bono* and the Popularization of Ficinian Platonism," in *Humanistica. Per Cesare Vasoli,* ed. Fabriziio Meroi and Elisabetta Scapparone (Florence: Leo S. Olschki, 2004), 61–69.
78. For definitions and caution against binaries, see Maxson, *Humanist World,* 10–11.
79. For the argument about humanism's impact, see ibid., 152; for discussion of the focus on politics and its limitations, see ibid., 63–64, 79–81, and 180.
80. Lynn Enterline, *Shakespeare's Schoolroom: Rhetoric, Discipline, Emotion* (Philadelphia: University of Pennsylvania Press, 2011).
81. Richard Palmer, *The Studio of Venice and Its Graduates in the Sixteenth Century* (Trieste: Edizioni LINT, 1983); Richard Palmer, "Nicolò Massa, His Family and His Fortune," *Medical History* 25 (1981): 385–410; Richard Palmer, "Pharmacy in the Republic of Venice in the Sixteenth Century," in *The Medical Renaissance of the Sixteenth Century,* ed. A. Wear, R. K. French, and I. M. Lonie (Cambridge: Cambridge University Press, 1985), 100–117; Gianna Pomata, *Contracting a Cure: Patients, Healers and the Law in Early-Modern Bologna* (Baltimore, MD: Johns Hopkins University Press, 1998); Katherine Park, *Doctors and Medicine in Early Renaissance Florence* (Princeton, NJ: Princeton University Press, 1985); Katherine Park, *Secrets of Nature: Gender, Generation and the Origins of Human Dissection* (Cambridge, MA: Zone Books of MIT Press, 2006).
82. David Gentilcore, *Healers and Healing in Early Modern Europe* (Manchester: Manchester University Press, 1998); Mary Lindemann, *Medicine and Society in Early Modern Europe* (Cambridge: Cambridge University Press, 1999).
83. Siraisi, *History, Medicine and the Traditions of Renaissance Learning*; See also Nancy Siraisi, "The Physician's Task: Medical Reputations in Humanist Collective Biographies," in *The Rational Arts of Living,* ed. A. C. Crombie and N. Siraisi (Northampton, MA: Smith College Department of History, 1987), 105–133, as well as Siraisi's analysis of the interpenetration of literary humanism

and the medical profession in physicians' academic and funerary orations in "Oratory and Rhetoric in Renaissance Medicine," *Journal of the History of Ideas* 65, no. 2 (2004): 191–211, and on physician-humanists' writings in diverse genres, "Medicine and the Renaissance World of Learning," *Bulletin of the History of Medicine* 78 (2004): 1–36.

84. Douglas Biow, *Doctors, Ambassadors, Secretaries: Humanism and the Professions in Renaissance Italy* (Chicago: University of Chicago Press, 2002); George McClure, *The Culture of Profession in Late Renaissance Italy* (Toronto: University of Toronto Press, 2004).

85. James Cushman Davis, *A Venetian Family and Its Fortune, 1500–1900: The Donà and the Conservation of Their Wealth* (Philadelphia: American Philosophical Society, 1975), xx. While Davis does concede that education helped members of the Donà family get government posts (12 and 52–54), education and culture play no larger role in the analysis. See also David Herlihy, "Three Patterns of Social Mobility in Medieval History," *Journal of Interdisciplinary History* 3, no. 4 (1973): 623–647; Dennis Romano, *Patricians and Popolani: The Social Foundations of the Venetian Renaissance State* (Baltimore, MD: Johns Hopkins University Press, 1987); Anna Esposito, "'Li nobili huomini di Roma': Strategie familiari tra città, Curia e municipio," in *Roma capitale: 1447–1527,* ed. Sergio Gensini (San Miniato, 1994), 373–388; and, most recently, John Padgett, "Open Elite?: Social Mobility, Marriage, and Family in Florence, 1282–1494," *Renaissance Quarterly* 63, no. 2 (2010): 357–411.

86. Maxson, *Humanist World,* 60–64, 79–81, 151, and 180.

87. Ibid., 84 and 173–176.

88. Dana Sajdi, *The Barber of Damascus: Nouveau Literacy in the Eighteenth-Century Ottoman Levant* (Stanford, CA: Stanford University Press, 2013).

89. Christopher S. Celenza, "Creating Canons in Fifteenth-Century Ferrara," *Renaissance Quarterly* 57, no. 1 (2004): 43–98; on humanists' testaments and hopes for posthumous honor, see 46–52.

90. Pierre Hadot, *The Inner Citadel: The* Meditations *of Marcus Aurelius,* trans. Michael Chase (Cambridge, MA: Harvard University Press, 2001), especially 48–51.

91. Matthew Lundin, *Paper Memory: A Sixteenth-Century Townsman Writes His World* (Cambridge, MA: Harvard University Press, 2012).

1. VENICE'S READING PUBLIC

1. Brian Maxson, *The Humanist World of Renaissance Florence* (Cambridge: Cambridge University Press, 2013).

2. Margaret L. King, *Venetian Humanism in the Age of Patrician Dominance* (Princeton, NJ: Princeton University Press, 1986); Craig Kallendorf, *Virgil and the Myth of Venice: Books and Readers in the Italian Renaissance* (Oxford: Clarendon Press, 1999); Patricia Brown, *Private Lives in Renaissance Venice: Art, Architecture and the Family* (New Haven, CT: Yale University Press, 2004).

3. Outstanding studies of notarial culture and testamentary practices are Maria Pia Pedani Fabris, *"Veneta auctoritate notarius": storia del notariato Veneziano (1514–1797)* (Milan: Giuffrè, 1996); Laurie Nussdorfer, *Brokers of Public Trust: Notaries in Early Modern Rome* (Baltimore, MD: Johns Hopkins University Press, 2009).
4. We find, for instance, stern injunctions against superfluity in one of the leading treatises on the notarial art circulating in the Veneto, Francesco Mantica's *Tractatus de coniecturis ultimarum voluntatem in libros XII distinctus* (Frankfurt: Martin Lechler for Sigmund Feyerabend, 1580), to which we will return in Chapter 2.
5. See especially Ronald Witt, "What Did Giovanni Read and Write? Literacy in Early Renaissance Florence," *I Tatti Studies in the Renaissance* 6 (1995): 83–114; Paul F. Grendler, *Schooling in Renaissance Italy: Literacy and Learning, 1300–1600* (Baltimore, MD: Johns Hopkins University Press, 1989); Robert Black, *Education and Society in Florentine Tuscany: Teachers, Pupils and Schools, c.1250–1500* (Leiden: Brill, 2007), 1–42; Kallendorf, *The Myth of Venice.* For literacy among the middling sort even earlier, see Armando Petrucci, *Writers and Readers in Medieval Italy: Studies in the History of Written Culture,* ed. and trans. Charles M. Radding (New Haven, CT: Yale University Press, 1995).
6. Susan Connell, "Books and Their Owners in Venice, 1345-1480," *Journal of the Warburg and Courtauld Institutes* 35 (1972): 163-186; Isabella Cecchini, "Collezionismo e mondo materiale," *Il collezionismo d'arte a Venezia* 2 (2008): 165-191; Marino Zorzi, "La circolazione del libro a Venezia nel Cinquecento: biblioteche private e pubbliche," *Ateneo veneto* 177 (1990): 117-189.
7. Cecchini discusses her findings for books in one paragraph in "Collezionismo," 178.
8. Ibid., 186, table 8.
9. Zorzi, "Circolazione," 128–129.
10. In an article cresting seventy pages, Zorzi devotes eight to everyday collectors; see ibid., 122–129.
11. Conservative estimates derive from Grendler, *Schooling in Renaissance Italy;* following him, Brian Richardson, *Printing, Writers and Readers in Renaissance Italy* (Cambridge: Cambridge University Press, 1999), esp. 109–112; optimistic figure derives from Black, *Education and Society,* 1–42. For an excellent survey of the topic and its discontents, see R. A. Houston, *Literacy in Early Modern Europe: Culture and Education 1500–1800* (London: Longman, 1988). David Cressy has also offered an intriguing state of the field essay treating the case of England in "Literacy in Context: Meaning and Measurement in Early Modern England," in *Consumption and the World of Goods,* ed. John Brewer and Roy Porter (London: Routledge, 1993), 305–319, which affirms the usual procedure of counting those able to sign their own names and yields rates of full literacy circa 1650 at less than 30 percent for men and less than 10 percent for women (see 305; for sliding scale of illiteracy broken down by group affiliation, see 315). Cressy does, however, problematize the different meanings (if not the

numbers) of literacy. Crucial, as these figures are difficult to square with the broad distribution of seventeenth-century and early eighteenth-century book owners elucidated by Lorna Weatherill in the same volume (206–227).

12. Grendler, *Schooling in Renaissance Italy.*
13. For the constrictions that Counter-Reformation culture placed on Venetian printing, see Paul F. Grendler, *The Roman Inquisition and the Venetian Press, 1540–1605* (Princeton, NJ: Princeton University Press, 1977).
14. Jane Bernstein, *Music Printing in Renaissance Venice: The Scotto Press, 1539–1572* (Oxford: Oxford University Press, 1998), 44–45.
15. For an excellent introduction to the perils and promises of Venetian household inventories, see Chriscinda Henry, "What Makes a Picture? Evidence from Sixteenth-Century Venetian Property Inventories," *Journal of the History of Collections* 23, no. 2 (2011): 253–265; for remarks on five as a point of demarcation between an assortment and a distinctive collection, see 256.
16. Zorzi, "Circolazione"; Albert Labarre, *Le livre dans la vie amiénoise du seizième siècle: L'enseignement des inventaires après décès, 1503–1576* (Paris: Nauwelaerts, 1971); Christian Bec, *Les livres des Florentins, 1413–1608* (Florence: Leo S. Olschki, 1984); Christian Bec, *Les marchands écrivains. Affaires et humanisme à Florence, 1375–1434* (Paris: Mouton, 1967). For good synthetic treatments of Italian book culture in particular, see Richardson, *Printing, Writers and Readers,* 118–121. And for a good recent survey of books in Venice, Marino Zorzi, "Le biblioteche veneziane, espresione di una singolare civiltà," in *The Books of Venice/Il libro veneziano,* ed. Lisa Pon and Craig Kallendorf (Venice: La musa Talìa and Oak Knoll Press, 2007), 1–31.
17. Zorzi, "Circolazione," 129.
18. Ibid., 121 and 126.
19. Bernardo Zonca (1528), ASV, Cancelleria Inferiore, Miscellanea Notai Diversi, Inventari, B.34, n.76. (Hereafter ASV, CI).
20. Catharina Raffono (1545), ASV, CI, B.37, n.43.
21. Vincenzo de Francesco (1579), ASV, CI, B.42, n.13.
22. Antonio (1576), ASV, CI, B.42, n.10.
23. Virginia Reinburg, *French Books of Hours: Making an Archive of Prayer, c.1400–1600* (Cambridge: Cambridge University Press, 2012). For that matter, eruditi read their texts wearing sometimes surprising sets of spectacles; see especially Lisa Jardine and Anthony Grafton, "Studied for Action: How Gabriel Harvey Read His Livy," *Past and Present* 129 (1990): 30–78.
24. Zorzi notes, but does not draw any larger significance, from similar occurrences of small but literary collections; see "Circolazione," 121.
25. Zuanne de Torre (1529), ASV, CI, B.34, n.88; Sabastiano Usnaghi (1578), ASV, CI, B.42, n.18; Pietro de Andrea (1589), ASV, CI, B.43, n.2.
26. Giorlamo Corner (1617), ASV, Giudici di Petizion, Inventari, B.346/11, n.114. (Hereafter ASV, GP.)
27. Nicolò Dolfin (1526), ASV, CI, B.34, n.24; Alvise Gradenigo (1538), ASV, CI, B.36, n.63; Pietro Gritti (1557), ASV, CI, B.39, n.59.

28. Richardson, *Printing, Writers and Readers,* 120.
29. Figure on wages derives from Frederic Lane, *Venice Maritime Republic* (Baltimore, MD: Johns Hopkins University Press, 1973), 333.
30. Leonardo Masser (1538), ASV, CI, B.36, n.71; Sebastiano Bordonio (1572), ASV, CI, B.42, n.49; Steffano Pozzo (1585), ASV, GP, B.338/3, n.69; Giacomo Grataruol (1587), ASV, CI, B.43, n.12; Steffano di Cerchieri (1584), ASV, CI, B.43, n.12.
31. Zuanne Alvise Bragadin (1566), ASV, CI, B.40, n.45; Hortensio Mulo (1590), ASV, CI, B.43, n.58; Christoffolo Vento (1583), ASV, GP, B.338/3, n.30; G[iovanni] Costa (1527) ASV, CI, B.34, n.46; Giovanni Battista Campanato (1555), ASV, CI, B.39, n.49; Alessandro de Gelo (1560), ASV, CI, B.40, n.64.
32. For an excellent analysis of Venetian furniture and decoration, see Patricia Fortini Brown, *Private Lives in Renaissance Venice: Art, Architecture and the Family* (New Haven, CT: Yale University Press, 2004).
33. Benedetto Superantio (1563), ASV, CI, B.40, n.17; Paolo Signa (1553), ASV, CI, B.38, n.64; Francesco de Maphei (1548), ASV, CI, B.38, n.17; Maria Vinciverre (1561), ASV, CI, B.40, n.71.
34. Francesco Livello (1527), ASV, CI, B.34, n.35.
35. Ibid.; Giacomo Pantaleo (1600), ASV, CI, B.45, n.5; Bernardino Redaldi (1527), ASV, CI, B.34, n.32.
36. Pamela Smith, *The Body of the Artisan: Art and Experience in the Scientific Revolution* (Chicago: University of Chicago Press, 2004).
37. James Amelang, *The Flight of Icarus: Artisan Autobiography in Early Modern Europe* (Stanford, CA: Stanford University Press, 1998).
38. James R. Farr, *Artisans in Europe, 1300–1914* (Cambridge: Cambridge University Press, 2000).
39. See especially Lauro Martines, *The Social World of the Florentine Humanists, 1390–1460* (Toronto: University of Toronto Press, 2011), esp. 6–12, 31, 198, 261–262, and 329.
40. Patrick Wallis, "Consumption, Retailing and Medicine in Early Modern London," *Economic History Review* 61, no. 1 (2008): 26–53.
41. W. David Kingerly, "Painterly Maiolica of the Italian Renaissance," *Technology and Culture* 34, no. 1 (1993): 28–48, esp. 37–39.
42. Bec, *Les marchands écrivains,* 407–415. Discussed in Petrucci, *Writers and Readers,* 186.
43. Richardson, *Printing, Writers and Readers,* 120.
44. Zorzi finds that only 26 percent of the patrician inventories he located refer to books and in many those constituted only a handful of volumes; see "Circolazione," 117–120.
45. Alvise Zorzi (1553), ASV, CI, B.38, n.71.
46. Catharina, widow of Ser Castelino (1571), ASV, CI, B.41, n.62.
47. Adrian Vidal (1577), ASV, CI, B.42, n.6: "libri de diverse sorte numero sessanta."
48. Adrian Vidal (1577), ASV, CI, B.42, n.6; Gerolemo a Solimatis (1560), ASV, CI, B.40, n.44; Angilberto Alemani (1564), ASV, CI, B.40, n.56.
49. Zorzi de Agaziis (1560), ASV, CI, B.40, n.72.

50. Alvisa Bonadia (1583), ASV, CI, B.43, n.3.
51. Andrea Marconi (1568), ASV, CI, B.41, n.15; Giuseppe Zarlino (1590), ASV, CI, B.43, n.16.
52. Zorzi de Antibaro (1549), ASV, CI, B.38, n.44.
53. Benedetto Premareno (1530), ASV, CI, B.35, n.9.
54. Zuanne Argentini (1533), ASV, CI, B.35, n.60.
55. Zuanne Battista Licino (1568), ASV, CI, B.41, n.22.
56. Antonio Abbardi (1644), IRE, DER E, B.137, fasc.1, fols.24v–27v.
57. A typical case is Francesco Gratiolo, who died in 1601, owned forty-three books, of which twenty related to his occupation (ASV, CI, B.45, n.21).
58. Francesco Livello (1527), ASV, CI, B.34, n.35.
59. Andrea Benivoli (1555), ASV, CI, B.39, n.15.
60. Alberto Quattrocchi inventory (1624), ASV, GP, B.349, n.25; Alberto Rini inventory (1604), Archivio IRE, DER E, B.189, fasc.3, n.30.
61. Marcantonio de Noale (1540), ASV, CI, B.37, n.29.
62. Ippolito Ganason (1584), ASV, GP, B.338/3, n.61.
63. Lodovico Usper (1601), ASV, GP, B.342/7, n.26.
64. Zampiero de Alessandri (1592), ASV, CI, B.44, n.40.
65. Florio Audet (1563), ASV, CI, B.40, n.14.
66. Paolo, q. Agustin (1574), ASV, CI, B.42, n.41.
67. Giacomo de Pergo (1538), ASv, CI, B.36, n.58.
68. Connell, "Books and Their Owners," 163–186.
69. Ibid., 163.
70. For mention of physicians, see Zorzi, "Circolazione," 125 (general) and 143–146 (discussion of Tomaso Rangone's attempt at a public library); for Guilandino di Marienburgo's 1589 bequest, see 149 and 153–154.
71. Zorzi does not tabulate numbers of volumes across categories; he included inventories with even one book, which skews the numbers downward.
72. Grendler, *Schooling in Renaissance Italy,* 43.
73. Ibid., 44–47.
74. Black, *Education and Society,* 1–42.
75. Petrucci, *Writers and Readers;* for Trecento Italy and the different literacies of the middling sort, see especially 148–189.
76. For a compelling new approach to understanding the mechanisms of that humanist entrenchment, see Maxson, *Humanist World of Renaissance Florence.*
77. Zorzi, "Circolazione," esp. 134.
78. Paul Grendler has found, for instance, only one case in Venice of a bookseller executed for peddling "prohibited books" (and the man in question, coincidentally named Pietro or Piero Longo, was likely also an unrepentant Protestant); see Grendler's *Roman Inquisition,* 186–189.
79. Bec, *Les livres des Florentines.*
80. Ibid., 124.
81. Renata Ago, *Il gusto delle cose. Una storia degli oggetti nella Roma del Seicento* (Rome: Donzelli Editore, 2006), 185–214.

82. For numerical summary, see ibid., 185; for breakdown by genre, see ibid., 193–201.
83. Albert Labarre, *Le livre dans la vie amiénoise du seizième siècle: L'enseignement des inventaires après décès 1503–1576* (Paris: Nauwelaerts, 1971), esp. 128–129 and 164–177. For discussion and reassessment, see Reinburg, *French Books of Hours,* 46 and 49–52.
84. For this argument, see especially Roger Chartier, *The Cultural Uses of Print in Early Modern France,* trans. Lydia Cochrane (Princeton, NJ: Princeton University Press, 1987). Yet Chartier does posit that the lines between vernacular and Latinate (or "popular" and "elite") reading practices have often been overdrawn, for instance, in Miriam Chrisman, *Lay Culture, Learned Culture: Books and Social Change in Strasbourg, 1480–1599* (New Haven, CT: Yale University Press, 1982).
85. Christiane Klapisch-Zuber, "The Name 'Remade': The Transmission of Given Names in Florence in the Fourteenth Century," in *Women, Family and Ritual in Renaissance Italy,* trans. Lydia Cochrane (Chicago: University of Chicago Press, 1985), 283–309; Sharon Strocchia, "Naming a Nun," in *Society and Individual in Renaissance Florence,* ed. William Connell (Berkeley: University of California Press, 2002), 215–240. See also David Herlihy, "Tuscan Names, 1200–1530," *Renaissance Quarterly* 51 (1988): 561–582.
86. ASV, Corpus Domini, B.2, "Corpus Dni. Domenicane," incipit "NOI GIOVANNI BADOARDO per Divina Misericordia Patriarca di Ven.a e Primate della Dalmatia," regulation 11. On the significance of naming more generally, see Strocchia, "Naming a Nun."
87. Will of Placido Ragazzoni (June 1, 1570), ASV Notarile Testamenti (Atti Secco), B.1192, n.544: "In oltre avendo io un figliolo bastardo in anverssa batizato con il nome di Beneto et poi pentitomi che il nome di nostro padre chadesi in figlioli non legitimi, me missi a nominarlo Scipione et cosi e continuato e continua adimandarsi."
88. Ibid., "il qualle figliolo e stato et e mio desiderio che atendi a le lettere acioche per quela via se faci un vuomo."
89. If Longo's daughter had been born much later, she might have been named for Saint Virginia, but that canonization did not happen until the later sixteenth century.
90. Will of Valerio Superchio (1540), ASV Notarile Testamenti (Atti Canal), B.191, n.672.
91. Will of Scipione Rini (1588), IRE DER E, B.189, fasc.1, n.36 (as marked).
92. ASV Notarile Testamenti (Atti Bianco), B.81, n.966.
93. Will of Ottavian Monaldi (1560), ASV Notarile Testamenti (Atti Bianco), B.81, n.837.
94. ASV Notarile Testamenti (Atti Cavanis), B.196, n.519.
95. ASV Notarile Testamenti (Atti Bianco), B.79, n.494.
96. Will of Faustina Fontana (1533), ASV Notarile Testamenti (Atti Zambelli), B.1101, n.105.

97. Will of Anzelica Baranzon (1548), ASV Notarile Testamenti (Atti Bianco), B.78, n.135.
98. These names are culled from several different sources: Adrian Vidal's household inventory, ASV, CI, B.42, n.6 and n.6bis; the 1591 autograph will of Letizia (or Cecilia) Vidal, ASV, Notarile Testamenti, B.222, n.1193; and the 1582 will of Lelio Vidal, ASV, Notarile Testamenti, B.222, n.1167.
99. Will of Cornelia, fu Francesco, moglie di Alexandro; ASV, Notarile Testamenti (Atti Bianco), B.79, n.270.
100. ASV Notarile Testamenti (Atti Michieli), B.646, n.346.
101. ASV Notarile Testamenti (Atti Cavanis), B.196, n.793.
102. ASV Notarile Testamenti (Atti Michieli), B.646, n.564; ASV Notarile Testamenti (Atti Bianco), B.80, n.512.
103. Will of Cecilia Vidal (June 22, 1591), ASV Notarile Testamenti (Atti Crivelli), B.222, n.193.

2. TESTAMENTARY HUMANISM

1. Stanley Chojnacki, "The Power of Love: Wives and Husbands in Late Medieval Venice," in *Women and Power in the Middle Ages,* ed. Mary Erler and Maryanne Kowaleski (Athens: University of Georgia Press, 1988); Stanley Chojnacki, *Women and Men in Renaissance Venice* (Baltimore, MD: Johns Hopkins University Press, 2000); Caroline Castiglione, "Accounting for Affection: Battles between Aristocratic Mothers and Sons in Eighteenth-Century Rome," *Journal of Family History* 25 (2000): 405–431.
2. Israel Abrahams, ed., *Hebrew Ethical Wills* (Philadelphia: Jewish Publication Society, 2006); Mark Cohen, ed. and trans., *The Autobiography of a Seventeenth-Century Rabbi: Leon of Modena's* Life of Judah, 2nd ed. (Princeton, NJ: Princeton University Press, 1989), 48, 55–57, and 174–178; and Natalie Zemon Davis, "Fame and Secrecy: Leon Modena's *Life* as an Early Modern Autobiography," also in the Cohen volume, 50–70.
3. Christopher S. Celenza, "Creating Canons in Fifteenth-Century Ferrara," *Renaissance Quarterly* 57, no. 1 (2004): esp. 46–52. For another instance, Coluccio Salutati's book bequests, see Armando Petrucci, *Writers and Readers in Medieval Italy: Studies in the History of Written Culture,* ed. and trans. Charles M. Radding (New Haven, CT: Yale University Press, 1995), 216–217.
4. Celenza, "Creating Canons," 52.
5. Will of Father Federico Leon, ASV Notarile Testamenti (Cavanis), B.194, n.451.
6. Anthony Grafton and Joanna Weinberg, *"I Have Always Loved the Holy Tongue": Isaac Casaubon, the Jews and a Forgotten Chapter in Renaissance Scholarship* (Cambridge, MA: Belknap Press of Harvard University Press, 2011), esp. chap. 5.
7. Will of Father Francesco, q. Zorzi (1563), ASV Notarile Testamenti (Cicrigni), B.199, n.280.
8. Will of Father Luca de Zorzi, ASV Notarile Testamenti (Cicrigni), B.199, n.474.

9. Will of Father Giovanni Solerio, ASV Notarile Testamenti (Secco), B.1192, n.454.
10. Will of Father Thomaso Fontana, ASV Notarile Testamenti (Bianco), B.81, n.955.
11. Will of Father Zorzi de S. Michiel, ASV Notarile Testamenti (Bianco), B.79, n.434.
12. Will of Symone dells Flossigliera, Parisien, ASV Notarile Testamenti (Bianco), B.81, n.929.
13. Will of Camillo Donà (1593), IRE, DER E, B.85, fasc. 1.
14. Will of Vettor Marcello (1584), ASV Notarile Testamenti (Secco), B.1192, n.602: "con i sui proprii danari guadagnasi nelli sui offitii ha comprato oltra i suoi drapi, vesti, fodri, libri, et ornamenti del suo studio li dui pera de cavadoni de bronzo [and a long list of other furniture] . . . dechiaro che de t[utt]e surrobe sono sue proprie dele quali non ha daffar alcuna divisione."
15. For parallel cases among modern elites, see Pierre Bourdieu, *Distinction: A Social Critique of the Judgement of Taste*, trans. Paul Kegan (London: Routledge, 1986), 84. For a contrasting view, emphasizing the strong cultural commitments of patricians, see Paula Findlen, "Ereditare un museo: Collezionismo, strategie familiari e pratiche culturali nell'Italia del XVI secolo," *Quaderni Storici* 115 (2004): 45–81.
16. Will of Paolo Pincio, ASV Notarile Testamenti (Secco), B.1192, n.538: "L'anno de la mia età Cinquantesimo settimo, & l'animo non meno per i molti et travagliosi pensieri, senza i quali non puo stare la vita nostra, stracco; che il corpo per le continue vigilie et fatiche di studii, consumato."
17. Will of Helena Usper, ASV Notarile Testamenti (Cavanis), B.194, n.356.
18. Will of Laura Codega, ASV Notarile Testamenti (Michiel), B.646, n.511.
19. Samuel Cohn, *Death and Property in Siena, 1205–1800* (Baltimore, MD: Johns Hopkins University Press, 1988).
20. Findlen, "Ereditare un museo," 53–59; Sarah Gwyneth Ross, *The Birth of Feminism: Woman as Intellect in Renaissance Italy and England* (Cambridge, MA: Harvard University Press, 2009), 53–94.
21. Pincio Will: "Voglio che sia Felippo, mio dilettissimo et dolcissimo figliuolo, havuto di Donna Crestina, donna di qualificati costumi, nell'ultima quasi età mia, piu per veder successor de la famiglia mia, come è natural desiderio, che per apitito voluptuoso. Et o figliuolo finalmente che sia o no, voglio che sia mio heriede, come ho ditto."
22. Ibid.: "Suplicando le lor. Es.e a pigliarlo in figliuolo proprio et quanto sara in loro operar' che si alievi nel timore di Dio et ne i studi"; "Finalmente attendj a i studij, ne i quali ti bisogna principalmente mantenere il nome di quella famiglia, de la quale sei restato solo et dal studio mio (il quale ti lascio per memoria de le mie vigilie) conosceraj che io ho acquistato, quello di che tu hora sei restato heriede, Perche ne da padre, ne da madre non ho mai havuto altro che l'essere . . . Dunque se tu ancora studieraj, haveraj honore et utile et finalmente a Dio et a gli homini saraj Caro."
23. Will of Nicolo Paruta, ASV Notarile Testamenti (Marsilio), B.1211, n.850.

24. Will of Placido Ragazzoni, ASV Notarile Testamenti (Secco), B.1192, n.544: "il qualle figliolo e stato et e mio desiderio che atendi a le letere acioche per quela via se faci un vuomo."
25. See especially Valeria Finucci, *The Manly Masquerade: Masculinity, Paternity and Castration in the Italian Renaissance* (Durham, NC: Duke University Press, 2003). Finucci's analysis does, however, helpfully situate masculinity, like femininity, as a performance.
26. Paradigm-shifting studies that present masculinity as contested include Mark Breitenberg, *Anxious Masculinity in Early Modern England* (Cambridge: Cambridge University Press, 1996); Michael Rocke, *Forbidden Friendships: Homosexuality and Male Culture in Renaissance Florence* (Oxford: Oxford University Press, 1998).
27. See Gadi Algazi, "Scholars in Households: Refiguring the Learned Habitus, 1480–1550," *Science in Context* 16 (2003): 9–42; Guido Ruggiero, *Machiavelli in Love: Sex, Self, and Society in the Italian Renaissance* (Baltimore, MD: Johns Hopkins University Press, 2010); Christopher Celenza, "Honor: The Humanists of the Classic Era on Social Place," in *The Lost Renaissance: Humanists, Historians and Latin's Legacy* (Baltimore, MD: Johns Hopkins University Press, 2005), 115–133.
28. Will of Zuanne Farsina (1564), ASV Notarile Testamenti (Cicrigni), B.199, n.377: "Et ordeno chel ditto mio fiolo sia solicitato a mandar ad imparar, et farlo diventar homo da ben."
29. See especially Ronald Witt, "What Did Giovanni Read and Write? Literacy in Early Renaissance Florence," *I Tatti Studies in the Renaissance* 6 (1995): 83–114; Paul F. Grendler, *Schooling in Renaissance Italy: Literacy and Learning, 1300–1600* (Baltimore, MD: Johns Hopkins University Press, 1989); Robert Black, *Education and Society in Florentine Tuscany: Teachers, Pupils and Schools, c.1250–1500* (Leiden: Brill, 2007), 1–42; Craig Kallendorf, *The Myth of Venice: Books and Readers in the Italian Renaissance* (Oxford: Clarendon Press of Oxford University Press, 1999).
30. Witt, "What Did Giovanni Read and Write?," 95.
31. Paul Gehl, *A Moral Art: Grammar, Society and Culture in Trecento Florence* (Ithaca, NY: Cornell University Press, 1993).
32. Kallendorf, *Myth of Venice,* 30–81.
33. Petrucci, *Writers and Readers.*
34. Spinelli accounts, Archivio IRE, DER E, B.195, fasc. 4.
35. See especially Burke, *Anthropology,* 113.
36. Maxson, *Humanist World;* Biow, *Doctors, Ambassadors, Secretaries;* Elizabeth McCahill, "Finding a Job as a Humanist: The Epistolary Collection of Lapo da Castiglionchio the Younger," *Renaissance Quarterly* 57, no. 4 (2004): 1308–1345.
37. Will of Martini Testa, ASV Notarile Testamenti (Cicrigni), B.199, n.497.
38. Will of Andriana Cathanio (1573), ASV Notarile Testamenti (Bianco), B.78, n.9: "Voglio che Marco quel havemo al presente in casa per amor di Dio el sia

tenuto et vestito et che li sia fatto insegnar a lezer da ditto mio marido alqual li lo racommando per anni quatro o cinque."

39. Witt, "What Did Giovanni Read and Write?," 101.
40. Will of Giacomo Cotre, ASV Notarile Testamenti (Bianco), B.79, n.482.
41. Will of Francesco Brognol, ASV Notarile Testamenti (Chiodo), B.201, n.151.
42. Will of Valerio Superchio, ASV Notarile Testamenti (Girolamo Canal), B.191, n.672, fol.3r: "Io non intendo che in la mia heredita l'habbia a far cosa alcuna, et se lui intrasse in qualche frenetico come sogliono fare li cativi preti non li boni, che non stimando la poverta di fratelli, la eta minore, le graveze della lita, domandare la legitima, in questo caso se pur le leze mi fosseno contra, Io voglio chel [rifaccia?] li dinari che lui me ha speso in studio malamente in qualche suo vivere licentioso, che peggio non voglio dire per honor suo, che arivano alla soma de piu de cinquecento ducati In quatro anni. Item. Voglio chel mi refaza li dinari chio ho speso in le bolle deli soi beneficii che furono piu de dussento cinquanta" and "exhortandoli al tempo debito proseguire el studio determinato et vegnire a perfettione Zoe Tyberio al dottorato di medicina, Alexandro al dottorato di legge, laltro a quello che parera a esser piu inclinato."
43. Superchio will, fol.1r.
44. Ross, *Birth of Feminism,* chap. 2; Findlen, "Ereditare un museo."
45. Will of Maffeo dei Maffei, ASV Notarile Testamenti (Marsilio), B.1210, n.714.
46. Will of Maddalena Quattrocchi, ASV Notarile Testamenti (Brinis), B.158, n.709.
47. Will of Philippo, Ceroicho all'Insegna delle Doi Ocche, ASV Notarile Testamenti (Michiel), B.646, n.325.
48. Will of Francesco Sansovino, ASV Notarile Testamenti (Cavanis), B.194, n.456: "Ne voglio per conto alcuno esser condotto a processione per piazza, ne per nessuno altro luogo, non essendo questa ceremonia d'obligo, ne di precetto, ma pura pompa mondana, et vanità', come attesta Santo Agostino, et di cio ne prego strettamente i miei Commissarii."
49. First will of Francesco Longo (1552), ASV Notarile Testamenti, Atti Bianco, B.79, n.355; final will (1574), ASV Notarile Testamenti, Atti Longin, B.1200, n.51. On Plutarch in the Renaissance, see Marianne Pade, "Sulla Fortuna delle Vite di Plutarco nell'Umanesimo Italiano del Quattrocento," *Fontes* 1 (1998): 101–116; as well as Marianne Pade, *The Reception of Plutarch's Lives in Fifteenth-Century Italy,* 2 vols. (Copenhagen: Museum Tusculanum Press, University of Copenhagen, 2007).
50. See especially Abrahams, *Hebrew Ethical Wills*; Cohen, *Autobiography,* 48, 55–57, and 174–178.
51. Cohen, *Autobiography,* 174–175.
52. Chojnacki, "Power of Love"; Chojnacki, *Women and Men;* Castiglione, "Accounting for Affection"; Cohn, *Death and Property in Siena.*
53. The scholarly literature on medieval and early-modern self-writing is voluminous, but some helpful studies are Paul Zumthor, "Autobiography in the

Middle Ages?," *Genre* 6 (1973): 29–48; Thomas Mayer and Daniel R. Woolf, eds., *The Rhetorics of Life-Writing in Early Modern Europe: Forms of Biography from Cassandra Fedele to Louis XIV* (Ann Arbor: University of Michigan Press, 1995); and Ronald Bedford, Lloyd Davis, and Philippa Kelly, eds., *Early Modern Autobiography: Theories, Genres, Practices* (Ann Arbor: University of Michigan Press, 2006). See also Stephen Greenblatt, *Renaissance Self-Fashioning from More to Shakespeare* (Chicago: University of Chicago Press, 1980); John Martin, "Inventing Sincerity, Refashioning Prudence: The Discovery of the Individual in Renaissance Europe," *American Historical Review* 102 (1997): 1309–1342; John Martin, *Myths of Renaissance Individualism* (New York: Palgrave Macmillan, 2004).

54. See Margaret King, *Venetian Humanism in the Age of Patrician Dominance* (Princeton, NJ: Princeton University Press, 1986), 92–205.
55. Will of Giovanni Soliero, ASV Notarile Testamenti (Secco), B.1192, n.454.
56. Will of Leo de Nigris, ASV Notarile Testamenti (Michieli), B.646, n.497: "Et perche dal principio del mio nascimento son stato infina hora in amorevolezza in candidezza et fraternita con messer Lorenzo mio fratello, perho voglio pregar ditto mio fratello che de tutto quello ch' è corso e fatto tra nui sia contento di acquietarse et voglia accettar quel pocco della mia parte che lasso a lui."
57. A provocative recent study is Dale Kent, *Friendship, Love and Trust in Renaissance Florence* (Cambridge, MA: Harvard University Press, 2009).
58. Will of Maffeo dei Maffei, ASV Notarile Testamenti (Marsilio), B.1210, n.714: "Et quanto io posso gli prego vogliano amarsi, come si conviene a boni fratelli"; "prego Giovanni Francesco, li [i.e., Giovanni Antonio] presto la reverentia che n' maggior fratelli si conviene."
59. Will of Nicolò Massa (final version), ASV Notarile Testamenti (Cavanis), B.196, n.870: "prego che tuti tre insieme se debbano amar e viver in pace e amorevolezza, aiutandossi l'uno con l'altro da fratelli e sorella con la pace de Dio e di messer Jesu Xro."
60. See Christopher S. Celenza, ed., *Angelo Poliziano's* Lamia: *Text, Translation and Introductory Studies* (Leiden: Brill, 2010), esp. 38–40.
61. Massa Draft Will (1562), IRE, ZIT E, B.30, n.4, fol.23v: "non essendo io debitor de alcuno. Et quello che io li ho lassato essendo mio libero, et per mi aquistado, et ancho come o' ditto non son debitor de persona alcuna, sia chi esser si voglia, salvo che de il mio Sig. Iddio Eterno, dalla infinita bonta del quale cognosco haver havuto tutti li beni cosi dell'anima come del corpo et roba et faculta, mediante le mie grande et assidue fatiche."
62. Will of Nicolò Paruta, ASV Notarile Testamenti (Marsilio), B.1211, n.850: "Perche il caso a me accorso per la paterna negligentia mi fa cauto et e continuo stimulo che tardando nel istesso error non incorri ho determinato Io Nicolo Paruta fu de messer Andrea con lo agiuto del omnipotente iddio creator de tutte cose et causa prima de tutte cause, anzi il caso de la incerta morte a miseri mortali all'improvista mi arsalti far el mio testamento et ultima volonta, accio quei pochi beni di fortuna che con l'agiuto suo et la induxtria mia acquistai et con la parsimonia conservai in sinistrum non un-

dino, anzi che chi rimanerano doppo me come qui sotto ordinero possino galdendoli talhor ricordarsi delle fatiche mie et vigilie."

63. Will of pre Federico Leon, ASV Notarile Testamenti (Cavanis), B.194, n.451: "ho deliberato far questo testamento de quel poco che Dio mi ha conceso con la industria de le lettere humane insignando et celebrando."
64. Will of Paolo Pincio (1597), ASV Notarile Testamenti (Secco), B.1192, n.538: "L'anno de la mia età Cinquantesimo settimo, & l'animo non meno per i molti et travagliosi pensieri, senza i quali non puo stare la vita nostra, stracco; che il corpo per le continue vigilie et fatiche di studdi, consumato; mi ricorda, che non molto longato sia quel giorno, nel quale Iddio clementissimo mio signor, comandi, che di questo albergo mortale partendomi, finischi di esser tale, quale per opera sua, fin' hora son stato."
65. Ibid.
66. Will of Alvise Bognolo, ASV Notarile Testamenti (Longin), B.1200, n.15: "quel che desidero che sia de quel poco di sustantia che m'ho aquistato con honeste fatiche."
67. Will of Giovanni Battista Peranda, ASV Notarile Testamenti (Ziliol), B.1259, n.563: "et volendo che il mio havere, qual mi ritrovo, acquistato con il mio esercitio con molte fatiche et sudori sia impiegato dopo la mia morte secondo il mio volere."
68. Baldassare Castiglione, *Il cortegiano* (Venice: Domenico Giglio, 1587), sig.G3r.
69. See Heather Gregory, ed., *The Selected Letters of Alessandra Strozzi,* bilingual ed. (Berkeley: University of California Press, 1997). See also Ann Crabb, *The Strozzi of Florence: Widowhood and Family Solidarity in the Renaissance* (Ann Arbor: University of Michigan Press, 2000).
70. Aby Warburg, *The Renewal of Pagan Antiquity: Contributions to the Cultural History of the European Renaissance,* trans. David Britt (Los Angeles: Getty Research Institute for the History of Art and the Humanities, 1999); Ernst Cassirer, *The Individual and the Cosmos in Renaissance Philosophy* (Oxford: Blackwell Publishing, 1963); Erwin Panofsky, *Renaissance and Renascences in Western Art* (Stockholm: Almquist and Wiksell, 1965). See also Silvia Feretti, *Cassirer, Panofsky and Warburg: Symbol, Art and History* (New Haven, CT: Yale University Press, 1989).
71. Will of Lorenzo Donado, ASV Notarile Testamenti (Secco), B.1192, n.425: "Ma fa bisogno di Attendere alli studii et Al'acquisto delle buone lettere per intendere cossi utili precetti et Santissimi misterii della Santissima Messa, Poiche l'udirla et non intenderla e di cossi Minor fruto et benefitio Al'anime nostre . . . et sopra il tutto gardarti dal gioco di carte o dadi, perche da esso puo troppo fa il inc.tro seguir ogni ruina et Male, cossi ne l'honore, come nella faculta, et quel che importa piu l'anima . . . il tratenimento delli studii delle buone lettere, et qualche alt.a virtu di Musica . . . atendi a tratenimenti et piaceri honoreveli, lassando da parte il gioco, qual non fa per chi ha da perdere . . . ma piu tosto per chi non ha da perdere niente, perche chi non ha non puo perdere, et credilo a me, perche so quello ti dico, per l'esperientia ch'io ho de tanti anni, Et pratica posso dire de tutte le cose del Mondo."

72. Will of Marc'Antonio Zantani (1536), ASV Notarile Testamenti (Marsilio), B.1211, n.778: "Hieronymo mio carissimo fiol sii mantenuto ala scuola dele arte liberal fin a tanto chel vegni suficiente ne le lre. et si [faccia così con] ogni altro mascolo me nasesse . . . et similiter le fie siano educate cum qualli mazior costumj sara possibile."
73. Antonio di Francesco Diedo (1572), ASV Notarile Testamenti (Longin), B.1200, n.5: "Li faccino imparar boni costumi, lettere, et sopra il tuto il timor di Dio, et che non li lassino star a Venetia, ma li tengano le Accademie."
74. Francesco Mantica, *Tractatus de coniecturis ultimarum voluntatem in libros XII distinctus* (Frankfurt: Martin Lechler for Sigmund Feyerabend, 1580); "Vitium superfluitatis quomodo sit fugiendum," sigs. K3v–K4r.
75. Of these eight churchmen, six were parish priests; only two held more prestigious positions on the ecclesiastical ladder.
76. Wills of Nicolò Massa, Draft (1562), IRE, ZIT E, B.30, fasc.4; (1569) registered will, ASV (Cavanis), B.196, n.870; Will of Giovanni Battista Peranda (1585), ASV (Ziliol), B.1259, n.563; Will of Federico Leon (1576), ASV (Cavanis), B.194, n.451; Will of Paolo Pincio (1597), ASV (Secco), B.1192, n.538.
77. *Physicians:* Longo, 1552 and 1574; Valerio Superchio (1540), ASV (Canal), B.191, n.672; Martial Rota (1561), ASV (Bianco), B.80, n.750; Maffeo de' Maffei (1561), ASV (Marsilio), B.1210, n.714; Benedetto Rini (1563), IRE, DER E, B.189, fasc.1, n.14; Vettore Bonagente (1566/7), ASV (Alchier), B.12, n.222; Michele di Muti (1571), ASV (Longin), B.1200, n.134; Giovanni Battista Doglioni (1643), IRE, DER E, B.180, fasc.1. *Priests:* Thomaso Fontana (1540), ASV (Bianco), B.81, n.955; Giovanni Solerio (1597), ASV (Secco), B.1192, n.454. *Lawyers:* Nicolò Paruta (1544), ASV (Marsilio), B.1211, n.850 and Leo de Nigris (1559), ASV (Michiel), B.646, n.497. *Patrician:* Lorenzo Donado (1588), ASV (Secco), B.1192, n.425. *Merchant:* Symone Flossigliera (1558), ASV (Bianco), B.81, n.955. *Artisan:* Laura Codega (1582), ASV (Michiel), B.646, n.511.
78. *Physicians:* Longo, 1574; Massa; Rota; Rini; Bonagente; Doglioni; Giuseppe Moletti (1570), ASV (Michieli), B.646, n.441; Giovanni Battista Peranda (1585), ASV (Ziliol), B.1259, n.563. *Priests:* Leon; Pincio; and Luca de Zorzi (1556), ASV (Cicrigni), B.199, n.474; Francesco di Zorzi (1563), ASV (Cicrigni), B.199, n.280; Thomaso Fontana (1540), ASV (Bianco), B.81, n.955; Zorzi di Michiel (1551), ASV (Bianco), B.79, n.434; and Giovanni Soliero (1597), ASV (Secco), B.1192, n.454.
79. *Patricians:* Cammilo Donà (1593), IRE, DER E, B.85, fasc.1; Vettor Marcello (1584), ASV (Secco), B.1192, n.602. *Lawyers:* Nicolò Eritreo (1542), ASV (Bianco), B.81, n.833; Leo de Nigris (1559), ASV (Michiel), B.646, n.497. *Merchant:* Symone Flossigliera (1558), ASV (Bianco), B.81, n.929.
80. Superchio; Massa; Rota; Maffei; Rini; Bonagente; Muti; Peranda; Doglioni; and Laura Forscarini Peranda (m. Battista Peranda), 1587 will, ASV (Ziliol), B.1259, n.653; Maddalena Quattrocchi (m. Alberto Quattrocchi), 1598 will, ASV (Brinis), B.158, n.709.

81. *Artisans:* Philippo de Rocco (1583), ASV (Michiel), B.646, n.325; Laura Codega (1582), ASV (Michiel), B.646, n.511. *"Citizens":* Francesco Brognol (1530), ASV (Chiodo), B.201, n.151; Placido Ragazzoni (1570), ASV (Secco), B.1192, n.544. *Lawyers:* Paruta; and Helena Usper (m. Lodovico Usper), 1589 will, ASV (Cavanis), B.194, n.356. *Merchants:* Martini Testa (1572), ASV (Cicrigni), B.199, n.497; Zuanne Farsina (1564), ASV (Cicrigni), B.199, n.377; Giacomo Cotre (1555), ASV (Bianco), B.79, n.482. *Patricians:* Donado; Zantani; and Antonio Diedo (1572), ASV (Longin), B.1200, n.5. *Priests:* Leon; Pincio.
82. *Physicians:* Longo; Superchio; Massa; Maffei; Peranda; Alvise Bognolo (1576), ASV (Longin), B.1200, n.15. *Priests:* Leon; Pincio; Fontana; Soliero; and Raphael Spatari (1560), ASV (Bianco), B.81, n.929.
83. *Artisan:* Codega. *Lawyers:* Paruta; Sansovino; Nigris. *Merchants:* Flossigliera; and Nicholo Grifo (1576), ASV (Bianco), B.81, n.836. *Patricians:* Donado; and Zuanne da Leze (1550), ASV (Bianco), B.79, n.496; Francesco da Mosto (1600), ASV (Ziliol), B.1243, n.269.
84. Matthew Lundin, *Paper Memory: A Sixteenth-Century Townsman Writes His World* (Cambridge, MA: Harvard University Press, 2012), esp. 33.
85. Ibid., 48–63 and 77.

3. NICOLÒ MASSA, A SELF-MADE MAN OF LETTERS

1. Francesco Sansovino, *Delle cose notabili della città di Venetia* (Venice: Agostin Zopini & Nepoti, 1596), 2:124.
2. Ibid., 132.
3. Richard Palmer, "Nicolò Massa, His Family and His Fortune," *Medical History* 25, no. 4 (1981): 385–410.
4. One of Palmer's archival finds was Massa's twenty-four-folio draft will of 1562 (IRE ZIT E, B.30, fasc.4), but he could not undertake close analysis of that within his article.
5. Nancy Siraisi, *Communities of Learned Experience: Epistolary Medicine in the Renaissance* (Baltimore, MD: Johns Hopkins University Press, 2013), 17–20.
6. Massa draft will (1562), IRE, ZIT E, B.30, n.4, fol.23v: "non essendo io debitor de alcuno. Et quello che io li ho lassato essendo mio libero, et per mi aquistado, et ancho come o' ditto non son debitor de persona alcuna, sia chi esser si voglia, salvo che de il mio Sig. Iddio Eterno, dalla infinita bonta del quale cognosco haver havuto tutti li beni cosi dell'anima come del corpo et roba et faculta, mediante le mie grande et assidue fatiche."
7. Nicolò Massa, *Liber introductorius anatomiae* (Venice: Francesco Bindoni and Maphei Pasini, 1536), sig.A2r: "Solent plerunque boni coloni, & si, qui summa diligentia agriculturae student, optimis quibusque selectis fructibus hero oblatis, testatum apud illum facere fructuum pulcritudine, atque amenitate, quantum in agro colendo, ac conserendo, opere laborisque impenderint.

Quorum diligentia & officiis oblectatus Dominus, libentius, ac liberalius agriculturae necessaria impartiri solet, ut coloni commodius & campos conferere, & fructes meliores, atque uberiores sibi, ac suis parare possint. Idem in litteraria cultura mihi faciendum existimari, nam cum iamdiu rei medicinae operam navarim, litterariosque agros coluerim, in ipsis non insuaves fructus conservi."

8. Ibid.: "una [ref: anatomical dissection] cum quampluribus non solum medicis, verum & aliarum bonarum artium cultoribus. Inter quos magnificum virum ac doctissimum philosophum Hieronymum Marcellum tamquam fidum Achatem semper habui, cui promisi me scripturum libellum introductorium."
9. Ibid., sig. A2v: "Suscipe igitur Pater Beatissime hos meos labores hilari vultu, ut me ad litterariam culturam te annuente confirmatum, meliores posthac & copiosiores fructus tibi offerentem videas."
10. For understanding physicians' letters as hybrid texts, see Siraisi, *Communities of Learned Experience,* esp. 11–12.
11. Massa, *Epistolarum,* vol. 2, sig.A1v: "magnis altissimisque rebus tractandis maiorem eloquentiam exoptandam non esse, cum res maximae & sublimes, quae ab eleganti intellectu moliuntur, satis per se ornatae & cultae sint. Siquidem mentis elegantiam & pulchritudinem in optimo discursu, & firmis rationibus consistere omnes sapientes affirmant, quibus si verborum fucum addideris, fortasse multum de sua maiestate detrahes, quemadmodum evenire pulchris mulieribus solet: quae cum vultus suos coloribus pingere student, nihil augent, sed deturpant potius pulchritudinem."
12. Christopher Celenza, ed., *Angelo Poliziano's* Lamia: *Text, Translation and Introductory Studies* (Leiden: Brill, 2010).
13. For this larger problem, see Francesco Bausi, *Nec rhetor nec philosophus fonti, lingua e stile nelle prime opere latine di Giovanni Pico della Mirandola (1484–1487)* (Florence: L. S. Olschki, 1996).
14. Celenza, "Poliziano's *Lamia* in Context," in his edition of *Angelo Poliziano's* Lamia, 39.
15. Massa, *Epistolarum,* sig.A2r.
16. See Pietro Aretino, *Cortigiana,* trans. J. Douglas Campbell and Leonard G. Sbrocchi (Ottawa: Dovehouse Editions, 2003).
17. Niccolò Machiavelli, *Mandragola,* trans. Mera J. Flaumenhaft (Prospect Heights, IL: Waveland Press, 1981).
18. Nicolò Massa, *De febri pestilentiali* (1555), sig. A2r: "ut antiquorum scriptorum exemplum sequerer, qui consuevere sua scripta in lucem edere sub patrocinio alicuis (ut aiunt) Mecoenatis, quo & robur, & auctoritatem maiorem consequerentur."
19. Ibid.: "frater tuus Philippus Landtgravius quasi alter Achilles."
20. For the various techniques of self-fashioning as a "man of letters," see especially Lisa Jardine, *Erasmus: Man of Letters; The Construction of Charisma in Print* (Princeton, NJ: Princeton University Press, 1993).

21. Massa, *Epistolarum,* vol. 2, sig. XX4r: "Cum per tot annos antea a doctissimo viro Ioanne Bernardo Foeliciano patruo suo (Bernardine) literas graecas addiscerem, assidua consuetudo similitudoque studiorum tantum amorem inter nos conciliavit, ut nullus esset dies quo aut ego domum vestram non venirem."
22. See especially Nancy Siraisi, *History, Medicine and the Traditions of Renaissance Learning* (Ann Arbor: University of Michigan Press, 2007).
23. K. J. P. Lowe, *Nuns' Chronicles and Convent Culture in Renaissance and Reformation Italy* (Cambridge: Cambridge University Press, 2003), esp. 62–63. For more general claims about medical consilia as evidence of humanism, see Roberto Cardini and Mariangela Religiosi, eds., *Umanesimo e medicina: il problema dell'individuale* (Rome: Bulzoni, 1996).
24. Petrarch, *Invectives,* trans. David Marsh (Cambridge, MA: Harvard University Press, 2008), 73. For another discussion of Petrarch's attack on physicians, see George McClure, *The Culture of Profession in Late Renaissance Italy* (Toronto: University of Toronto Press), 8.
25. On physicians' incomes and honoraria, see Elena Brambilla, "La medicina del Settecento: dal monopolio dogmatico alla professione medica," in *Storia d'Italia, Annali 7 (Malattia e Medicina),* ed. Franco della Paruta (Turin: Einaudi, 1984), 133–147.
26. Nancy Siraisi, "The Physician's Task: Medical Reputations in Humanist Collective Biographies," in *The Rational Arts of Living* (Northampton, MA: Smith College Library, 1987), 105–133, esp. 120; McClure, *Culture of Profession,* 7–9, 110–115, and 195–200. See also George McClure, "The *Artes* and the *Ars moriendi* in Late Renaissance Venice: The Professions in Fabio Glissenti's *Discorsi Morali contra il dispiacer del morire, detto Athanatophilia* (1596)," *Renaissance Quarterly* 51, no. 1 (1998): 92–127.
27. On the fraught boundary between medical work as a "civil profession" and as manual labor, with attendant issues of social hierarchy and family origins, see Brambilla, "La medicina del Settecento," 6–10, 33–39, 137, and 145.
28. Tommaso Garzoni, *Piazza universale di tutte le professioni del mondo* (Venice: Roberto Meglietti, 1605), 152–161.
29. Fabio Glissenti, *Discorsi morali contra il dispiacer del morire, detto Athanatophilia* (Venice: Domenico Farri, 1596), 196r.
30. BNM, "Notizie," MS It. VII, 2342 (=9695), fol.82r.
31. James Hankins, *Plato in the Italian Renaissance* (Leiden: Brill Academic Publishing, 1990), especially 95ff. and 363; James Hankins, "Humanism in the Vernacular: The Case of Leonardo Bruni," in *Humanism and Creativity in the Renaissance: Essays in Honor of Ronald G. Witt,* ed. Christopher Celenza and Kenneth Gouwens (Leiden: Brill, 2006), 11–29.
32. Paul F. Grendler, *The Universities of the Italian Renaissance* (Baltimore, MD: Johns Hopkins University Press, 2002), esp. 140; Nancy Siraisi, *Medieval and Early Renaissance Medicine: An Introduction to Knowledge and Practice* (Chicago: University of Chicago Press, 1990), 18; A. Wear, R. K. French and I. M. Lonie, eds.,

The Medical Renaissance of the Sixteenth Century (Cambridge: Cambridge University Press, 1985), 80.

33. Richard Palmer, *The Studio of Venice and Its Graduates in the Sixteenth Century* (Trieste: Edizioni Lint, 1983), esp. 20–31 and 51. For the crack about "paper universities," see Grendler, *Universities,* 140.
34. Palmer, *Studio of Venice,* 41–43.
35. Siraisi, *History, Medicine and the Traditions*; Nancy Siraisi, "Medicine and the Renaissance World of Learning," *Bulletin of the History of Medicine* 78 (2004): 1–36; on the issue of "occupational diversity" specifically, see Sandra Cavallo and David Gentilcore's introduction to their edited volume, *Spaces, Objects and Identities in Early Modern Italian Medicine* (Oxford: Blackwell Publishing, 2008), 5–6. See also Margaret Pelling, "Occupational Diversity: Barber-Surgeons and the Trades in Norwich, 1550–1640," *Bulletin of the History of Medicine* 56 (1982): 484–511.
36. Siraisi, *History, Medicine and the Traditions,* 263.
37. Palmer, "Nicolò Massa," 386 and 406.
38. Alvise Luisin, *Dialogo intitolato la cecità* (Venice: Giorgio de' Cavalli, 1569), 10.
39. Ibid., 15 et seq.
40. Virginia Cox, The *Renaissance Dialogue: Literary Dialogue in Its Social and Political Contexts, Castiglione to Galileo* (Cambridge: Cambridge University Press, 1992).
41. Luisin, *Dialogo,* 19–21. Palmer views Apollonio as a Lutheran; Siraisi questions this interpretation in *Communities of Learned Experience,* 19.
42. Luisin, *Dialogo,* 38.
43. Ibid.
44. Pierre Hadot, *The Inner Citadel: The Meditations of Marcus Aurelius,* trans. Michael Chase (Cambridge, MA: Harvard University Press, 2001), 4–5, 76–77, 81–82, and 183–231; Christopher Celenza, "What Counted as Philosophy in the Italian Renaissance? The History of Philosophy, the History of Science and Styles of Life," *Critical Inquiry* 39, no. 2 (2013): 385.
45. Luisin, *Dialogo,* 38.
46. Nancy Siraisi, "Oratory and Rhetoric in Renaissance Medicine," *Journal of the History of Ideas* 65 (2004): 191–211. See also Siraisi, *History, Medicine and the Traditions,* esp. 113–119.
47. For Trincavella's reputation and the numbers of students, see Palmer, *Studio of Venice,* 19–20. The version of the oration I will be using in the following analysis is a MS transcription by Apostolo Zeno, BNM, MS It. VII, 351 (=8385), ff.350r–352v. Hereafter Castelli.
48. Castelli, fol.351r.
49. Castelli, fols.351r and 352r: "Qui sane vir doctissimus, cum iam ab omnibus magnus Phisicus et summus Theologus existimaretur, noluit tamen a musis poenitus, et disciplinis mathematicis abhorere. Itaque interdum Poetas et Historicos summa cum voluptate [legebat], Geometras, Arithmeticos, Musicos, Astrologos omnes in manibus saepe habebat, ut qui multorum lectione plurimum delectaretur, quasi vero omnem disciplinarum orbem cir-

cumplectendum sibi esse putaret." Here we see find the *grammaticus* and philosopher both expected to read broadly, a point reinforced in Celenza, *Angelo Poliziano's* Lamia, esp. 13 and 39.

50. Castelli, fol.351v: "Sed his summis dotibus non contentus hic vir vere ad bene merendum de hominibus quid quid temporis aut ocii sibi horis successivis [concessiderat] id omne in bonarum artium studiis excolendis iuvandisque posteris assidue, posuit ut quam ille scientiam summo labore acquiescerat, libentissime quoque aliis, et liberalissime communicaret."
51. Alberto Rini's "Giornali," ASV, Scuola Grande di San Marco, B.112, fasc. 1, memorandum in Giornale A, dated August 21, 1563: "Lo Ex.te messer Victor Trincavella medico mio compare che haveva lectura de pratica a Padoa et este sepulto . . . et messer Domenego de Castello fece la . . . oration la domenega."
52. Vettore Trincavella, *Opera omnia* (Lyons: Giunti & Paulo Guitto, 1586), sigs.+4r-+5r.
53. Siraisi, *History, Medicine and the Traditions,* 17.
54. Massa draft will, fol.14v: "Al qual Francesco lasso delli mei libri da studiar quanti ne vora lui, quali voglio li siano dati per Maria sua madre, et sia antiposto in questo a tutti li altri, et tora cosi volgari come latini, et greci in ogni sorta de scienza et arte che si troverano et besognandoli voglio si faccia dar quelli che havera havuto Lorenzo et Apollonio sui barbari, et questo senza alcuna contradicion et con contento de sua madre." For provisions regarding Apollonio's free use of his medical books, see this draft will, fol. 13v. For Massa's bequest of medical books to his professional protégé, Zuanne Grataruol, see the will he ultimately registered, ASV, Notarile Testamenti, Atti Marc'Antonio Cavanis, B.196, n.870, fol.2v.
55. Houshehold inventory of Maria Massa (1586), IRE ZIT E, B.29, fasc.8, fols. 13v and 15r–v: "una cassa segnata no.15: Libri a stampa de diverse sorte no. settantacinque" and "una meza cassa segnata no.Disdotto piena de libri a stampa et penna picioli et grandi."
56. Account Book of Nicolò Massa, IRE ZIT E, B.30, fasc.3.
57. On Mercuriale, see Siraisi, *History, Medicine and the Traditions,* esp. 42–55, 63–64, 183–186; on *De arte gymnastica* (which may be the volume indicated here), see 47–50 and 53. See also Nancy Siraisi, "History, Antiquarianism and Medicine: The Case of Girolamo Mercuriale," *Journal of the History of Ideas* 64, no. 2 (2003): 231–251.
58. For all these loans, see Account Book of Nicolò Massa, IRE ZIT E, B.30, fasc.3, fol.1v.
59. Quattrocchi inventory, ASV Giudici di Petizion, Inventari, B.349, n.25.
60. For analysis of this category and its changing boundaries, see Ann M. Blair, *Too Much to Know: Managing Scholarly Information before the Modern Age* (New Haven, CT: Yale University Press, 2010), 118–132.
61. On the wide range of "self-help" literature available in Renaissance Italy, see Rudolph Bell, *How to Do It: Guides to Good Living for Renaissance Italians* (Chicago: University of Chicago Press, 1999). On the art of memory, see Frances

Yates, *The Art of Memory* (Chicago: University of Chicago Press, 1966); Jonathan Spence, *The Memory Palace of Matteo Ricci* (New York: Penguin, 1985).

62. Paul F. Grendler, *The Roman Inquisition and the Venetian Press, 1540–1605* (Princeton, NJ: Princeton University Press, 1977), 186–187.
63. Peter Burke, *A Social History of Knowledge: From Gutenberg to Diderot* (Malden, MA: Polity Press, 2000), 170.
64. Anthony Grafton, *Commerce with the Classics: Ancient Books and Renaissance Readers* (Ann Arbor: University of Michigan Press, 1997).
65. See especially Margaret Meserve, *Empires of Islam in Renaissance Historical Thought* (Cambridge, MA: Harvard University Press, 2008); Lucette Valensi, "The Making of a Political Paradigm: The Ottoman State and Oriental Despotism," in *The Transmission of Culture in Early Modern Europe,* ed. Anthony Grafton and Ann Blair (Philadelphia: University of Pennsylvania Press, 1990), 173–203; Nancy Bisaha, *Creating East and West: Renaissance Humanists and the Ottoman Turks* (Philadelphia: University of Pennsylvania Press, 2004).
66. For early-modern historians' increasing professionalization in the sixteenth century, see Anthony Grafton, *What Was History? The Art of History in Early Modern Europe* (Cambridge: Cambridge University Press, 2007).
67. The inventory of books comprises part of the larger household inventory of the Rini family, IRE DER E B.189, fasc.3, n.30; for the books, see ff.6v–12r.
68. Giornali di Alberto Rini, ASV, Scuola Grande di San Marco, B.112, fasc.1, Giornale A (unfoliated, spanning the years 1557-1574) and Giornale B (foliated, spanning the years 1574–1599). Hereafter, I will refer to the journals as "Giornale A" and "Giornale B." On his books in Giornale A, see the entry dated September 1571 appearing at the end of the journal in a section of general notes.
69. Giornale B, fol.186v.
70. Rini's purchases by genre break down as follows: astrology (three volumes); biography (ten); classical authors (three); dictionaries and lexicons (six); epistles (three); history (twelve); medicine (four); contemporary literature, including poetry (three volumes); theology and devotion (fifteen volumes).
71. Susan Connell, "Books and Their Owners in Venice," *Journal of the Warburg and Courtauld Institutes* 35 (1972): esp. 177.
72. Albert Labarre, *Le livre dans la vie amiénoise du seizième siècle: L'enseignement des inventaires après décès (1503–1576)* (Paris: Nauwelaerts, 1971), esp. 128–129.
73. Palmer, "Nicolò Massa," 386.
74. IRE ZIT E, B.30, fasc.4.
75. Ibid., fol.1r: "Te Deum patrem omnipotentem et Hyesu. Xrm. filium tuum, et spiritum sanctum, unum Deum Eternum: tota mente suplex oro et preco ut mentem mea ilumines, et regas, nequod iniustum scribam aut inofficiosum, vel quod materia litigandi alicui prestare possit, in hoc meo ultimo testamento, et ultima voluntate; quod testamentum ut clarius intelligatur sit cum volgari sermone scribere incipiam."

76. On testators marking their confessional allegiances, see Samuel Cohn, *Death and Property in Siena, 1205–1800: Strategies for the Afterlife* (Baltimore, MD: Johns Hopkins University Press, 1988), 164–216.
77. Will of Valerio Superchio (1540), ASV, Notarile Testamenti (Canal), B.191, n.672: "Anchora che io sia professore de l[ette]re l'ho fatto in lingua materna a maggior Intelligentia de quelli che l'ho haveranno a veder et exequire."
78. See Sarah Gwyneth Ross, *The Birth of Feminism: Woman as Intellect in Renaissance Italy and England* (Cambridge, MA: Harvard University Press, 2009), chap. 1.
79. Massa draft will, fol.3r: "Item. mi tro haver beni mobeli de diverse sorte, trali quali vi sono arzenti et ori lavoradi zoglie annelli, Danari tapezarie et altri ornamenti diversi di casa, libri et altre mie cose che non nominaro de uno in uno."
80. Ibid., fol.13r: "li lasso al ditto Lorenzo per la medesima rason de heredita uno anneleto de oro qual ha una corniola ligada nella qual vi e intagliate alcune figure acavalo et a piedi, e si crede essere talio anticho." He crossed out this description in later deliberations.
81. On this multidimensional collecting, see Renata Ago, *Il gusto delle cose. Una storia degli oggetti nella Roma del Seicento* (Rome: Donzelli Editore, 2006).
82. Massa, fol.6r: "Maria lasso alla ditta maira tutti li mei beni mobelli che si trovaranno in casa mia o fuora de casa in quel luogo esser si voglia, et de qual sorta esser si voglia, nelli quali mobeli voglio se intenda cosi ori come arzenti, annelli, zoglie, et ogni altra sorte de ornamenti de studii camere [de casa che si troverano cosi nelle camere come nelli studii che sarano mie casse de ogni sorte]."
83. Ibid., fol.11v: "Item. Lasso a Apollonio ditto qual dalle fasse (fino al tempo si volse maridar cum Madonna Gratiosa fiola del qm. Nobile Homo messer Lorenzo di Martini advochato) Io lo tenuto in casa, nutrito, vestito et fato studiar in diversi studi, et fatosi dottor delle Arte et medicina, per le qual tutte cose ho speso per lui tutti deli mei molti et molti danari, oltra molte fatiche per mi fate, et molti affani et fastidii havuti per lui, delli quali spesi per lui deli mei danari, et datoli in diversi tempi deli quali alcuni ne ho notadi nelli mei libri et molti non sono notado quali non notadi sono molto più assai de quelli che io ho notadi, delli molti datoli et per lui spesi come in parte si portra veder per sue lettere a me scritto che haverli receputi, et anchora per lettere mi pregava li volesse mandarli denari, et ahcho per lettere de cambio pagato per lui, et altri spesi et diversi tempi delli quali tutti lui me è debitor, El qual tutto suo debito, et mio credito, cosi de prestandi come de spesi et pagati per lui il lasso per rason de heredita et per ogni altra causa pretension o rason che lui credesse dover haver da mi per qual se voglia modo."
84. Ibid.: "Lasso a Lorenzo Massa mio nepote fiolo de Paula mia sorella al qual Lorenzo io ho sempre et con ogni studio cercado de Zovarli con non pocha mia fatica et spesa facendoli insegnar boni costumi, et bone lettere, cosi nella cita come in Padoa et altrove, acio tandem venisse homo honorato per le sue proprie virtu come è venuto, Dico prima che li lasso ogni quantita de danari

spesi per lui et datoli per mi de contadi in diversi tempi, li quali cosi spesi come altri datti, alcuni io ho notadi nelli mei libri et molti non sono notadi, et sono molto piu che li notadi, Qual tutto suo debito et mio credito li lasso per rason de heredita et ogni altra causa o cosa che lui pretendesse dover haver da mi per qual si voglia rason."

85. Ibid., fols.13r–v: "Item. li lasso delli mei libri se ne havera bisogno per studiar quanti parara a Maria, la qual ne tenira conto et nota, de quanti ne havera dati, acioche poi bisognando quelli a Francesco suo fiol o altri sui fioli se ne havera come ho ditto overo se essa Maria li volesse per lei per quale si voglia causa, li possi rihaver, il tutto tamen voglio sia per conto de heredita, se ben bisognando li restituera. anchora voglio che se Apollonio havera bisogno de qualche uno delli ditti mei libri et massimo de medicina, li siano dati per Maria ditta la qual ne tenira conto de quanto ne havera datti, acioche se besognandoli li vora in drieto, oper lei o per sui fioli, possi farseli restituir, non pero voglio possi esser astretta ditta Maria a darli a qual si voglia de loro, se lei non vora, ma del tutto fara lei quanto li parera stia bene."
86. Ibid., fol.13v: "De Francesco fiolo de Maria quale io amo cordialissimamente et ho deffeso da tante insidie, et litte fatoli dalli sui parenti da parte de suo padre, non diro altro salvo che lo ricommando prima a dio nostro signore qual è primo protetor dei pupilli et vedove et poi a Maria sua madre, se ben so quanto lei anchora l'ama sapendo quante fatiche et incomodi, affani ha supportato per relevarlo. Dico che lo ricommando che continui a relevarlo nel timor et reverentia de Dio et nelli boni costumi, et lo faccia continuar neli boni studi de bone lettere et nelle virtu christiana."
87. Final will of Nicolò Massa, ASV Notarile Testamenti (Cavanis), B.196, n.870.
88. Ibid.: "Lasso alli sopraditti Maria mia fia e, messer Appollonio e messer Lorenzo mie nepoti e, commissarii tuti li mei libri, ma prima ditta Maria possi tuor fuora e ellezer qual sorte de libri Latini, o vulgari li parera."
89. Ibid.: "prego ditti mei Nepoti che vedano con diligentia se su essi libri ne fosse qualcheduno prohibito dalli Sacri Ordeni del Concilio, overa contra *bonos mores,* et trascandone, quelli tali siano brusati, over dessi sia fato quanto e ordinato per Il Sacro Santo Concilio."
90. On literary and intellectual culture's responses to Trent, see especially John O'Malley, *Trent and All That: Renaming Catholicism in the Early Modern Era* (Cambridge, MA: Harvard University Press, 2000); Grendler, *Roman Inquisition;* Diana Robin, *Publishing Women: Salons, the Presses and the Counter-Reformation in Sixteenth-Century Italy* (Chicago: University of Chicago Press, 2007); Virginia Cox, *The Prodigious Muse: Women's Writing in Counter-Reformation Italy* (Baltimore, MD: Johns Hopkins University Press, 2011).
91. Final will of Nicolò Massa: "Ordeno che ditti mie commissarii habbino a servir ditto messer Zuanne Grataruol delli mei libri de praticha de medicina che li facesse Bisogno, si come a loro commissarii parera."
92. Ibid.: "Ordeno che nella divisione delli libri che farano ditti mie Nevodi e fiola, Cadauno d'essi habbi a tuor le materia e volumi intieri e non smembrati,

I quali prego che tuti tre insieme se debbano amar e viver in pace e amorevolezza, Avitandossi l'uno con l'altro da fratelli e sorella con la pace de Dio e di messer Iesu Xro."

93. Will of Valerio Superchio (1540), ASV, Notarile Testamenti (Canal), B.191, n.672: "El residuo veramente de tutti li mei beni presente e futuri mobeli e stabeli lasso agli miei charissimi figlioili . . . exhortandoli al tempo debito proseguire al studio determinato et vegnire a perfettione Zoe Tyberio al dottorato di medicina, Alexandro al dottorato di legge."
94. Ibid.: "Lasso alle mie charissime figliole . . . in segno di amore ducati dese per una, le quale vero è che non hanno havuto quelle dote che meriteriano . . . per due rasone, prima perche non hanno bisogno, et per gratia de Iddio, sonno maritate di [sopra?], dove stanno honoratissimamente come se fussero signore, l'altra perche quando Io le maritai ero richo de animo et de honore, ma povero di roba, ne havevo oltra settanta ducati de intrada."
95. Ibid.
96. See household inventory of Maria Massa ZIT E 29, 8; on the Zitelle and Veronica Franco, see Margaret Rosenthal, *The Honest Courtesan: Veronica Franco, Citizen and Writer in Sixteenth-Century Venice* (Chicago: University of Chicago Press, 1993), 77, 129–134.
97. For this tangible monument, see Palmer, "Nicolò Massa."
98. Matthew Lundin, *Paper Memory: A Sixteenth-Century Townsman Writes His World* (Cambridge, MA: Harvard University Press, 2012).
99. Ibid., esp. 33–36 and 171–176.

4. FRANCESCO LONGO'S PHILOSOPHICAL TESTAMENTS

1. The 1574 will of Francesco Longo, ASV, Notarile Testamenti (Atti Longin), B.1200, n.51. Hereafter Longo, 1574.
2. Elda Martellozzo Forin, ed., *Acta gradum academicorum gymnasii Patavini ab anno 1526 ad annum 1537* (Padua: Editrice Antenore, 1970), 179–182 and 361–368.
3. The 1552 will of Francesco Longo, ASV, Notarile Testamenti (Atti Bianco), B.79, n.355. Hereafter Longo, 1552.
4. See Maria Pia Pedani Fabris, *"Veneta auctoritate notarius": storia del notariato Veneziano (1514–1797)* (Milan: Giuffrè, 1996), 100–101.
5. On notarial arts and processes, and the complex social and quasi-familial nature of the notary's role, see Laurie Nussdorfer, *Brokers of Public Trust: Notaries in Early Modern Rome* (Baltimore, MD: Johns Hopkins University Press, 2009).
6. Pietro Longo's doctorate is recorded as conferred on April 27, 1556, in the "Elenco Priori e Dottorati," BNM, MS It. VII, 2379 (=9896), fol.18v and as conferred on February 27 in "Notizie trade dai Libri dei Priori," BNM, MS It. VII, 2342 (=9695), fol.96r. On examinations, see Richard Palmer, *The Studio of Venice and Its Graduates in the Sixteenth Century* (Trieste: Edizioni LINT, 1983),

37. On Pietro Longo's blindness as of 1592 and exemption from the College's taxes as of that year, see 145.

7. Cornelio's (evidently unsuccessful) business enterprises, especially in real estate, emerge in the list of Pietro Longo's papers and accounts in the household inventory made after his death (1608), ASV, Giudici di Petizion, Inventari, B.343/8, n.93.

8. Longo, 1574: "Fra me medesimo spesse voler considerano, quello che da alcuno mai troppo et da pochissimi a bastanza è considerato, cioè del fine nostro, et della morte: qual pensiero, et cognitatione, ne superfluo puo essere, ne ancora troppo [testo] da alcuno considerato consciosia che la morte a tutti sia molto certissima, et l'hora di essa incertissima utile cosa, et honesta ho creduto esser a ciascuno delle cose sue deliberare, inanci, che la morte pervenghi; la quale per molti varij et diversi casi dubiosissimi delle cose nostre imminente pericolo ne minaccia, et a molti non pensandoli poco lontana da essi si ritrova ancora che giovanni siano, non che in etade senile, come son io, quale per gratia de Dio de anni sesantaotto sano del corpo, et della mente; di me medesmo et delle cose mie ho proposto voler ordinar' questa mia ultima volontade, benche per dir il vero cosi poche et piciole siano, che quasi mi vergogno di quelle mention farne per testamento. pur essendo gli pensieri delle lor cose, cosi de gli richi, come delli poveri, ancora che non eguali, nondimeno sono tutti dimandati pensieri."

9. Christopher Celenza, "What Counted as Philosophy in the Italian Renaissance? The History of Philosophy, the History of Science, and Styles of Life," *Critical Inquiry* 39 (2013): 367–401; for philosophy as a "style of life," see esp. 369, 385, and 398–399; Pierre Hadot, *The Inner Citadel: The* Meditations *of Marcus Aurelius* (Cambridge, MA: Harvard University Press, 2001), 4–5 and 190–191.

10. Margaret King, *Venetian Humanism in an Age of Patrician Dominance* (Princeton, NJ: Princeton University Press, 1986), 174–192.

11. The most comprehensive treatment of early-modern interactions with Plutarch is Marianne Pade, *The Reception of Plutarch's Lives in Fifteenth-Century Italy* (Copenhagen: Museum Tusculanum Press, University of Copenhagen, 2007). See also Marianne Pade, "Sulla Fortuna delle Vite di Plutarco nell'Umanesimo Italiano del Quattrocento," *Fontes* 1 (1998): 101–116; Christopher S. Celenza "'Parallel Lives': Plutarch's *Lives,* Lapo da Castiglionchio the Younger (1405–1438) and the Art of Italian Renaissance Translation," *Illinois Classical Studies* 22 (1997): 121–155; and Vito Giustiniani, "Sulle Traduzioni Latine delle 'Vite' di Plutarco nel Quattrocento," *Rinascimento* 1 (1961): 3–62.

12. Longo, 1574: "Io ho desiderato che in vita mia et dapoi la morte, voi tutti miei figlioli fusti de uno volere, et unanimi tra voi, considerando quello che Artaxerse famosissimo Re di Persi, fece essendo vicino alla morte sua, quale fattosi portar un gran mazzo di frece alla presentia de suoi figlioli, insieme tutti legate, a ciascuno delli detti le presenti, che insieme le spezassero gli comando, il che non possendo far alcuno de loro, gli disse . . . separate tutte

l'una dall'altra, le rompesserò, qualcosa prestissimo fu fatta da essi, et rotte, che furno tutte, al'hora disse Artaxerse, vedete figlioli, se voi sareti uniti, insieme, di valore, et di animo, e di forze niuno vi superata, ne spezzarà la potentia vostra, ma, se divisi sareti di volere, potrete presto esser suparati, et vinti da vostri nemici, come . . . avete veduto."

13. I thank Jill Kraye for helping me to sort out Longo's misattribution.
14. Plutarch, "De garulitate," in *Moralia VI, 511C,* trans. W. C. Helmbold (Cambridge, MA: Harvard University Press, 1939).
15. On Renaissance interactions with Plutarch's "Life of Artaxerxes" specifically, see Pade, *Reception,* 1:292–299 and 2:157–164; Celenza, "Parallel Lives," 133–134.
16. On Plutarch texts in patronage and friendship economies, see again Celenza, "Parallel Lives"; Pade, *Reception,* 1:27 and 185–187; 2:297–299.
17. Longo, 1552: "Et in segno di amor lasso al dicto Messer Girardo mio fradello el mio annello da bolla qual voglio che lo galdi per amor mio, pregandolo che lacetti piu la mia ben volonta che il presente aricordandoli che Artaserse famosissimo Re di Persia non hebbe a sdegno gustar le cristalline aque dal tralucido fonte tolto dalle cullose mani di uno rozzo villano considerando l'affetto et non l'effetto del bever de l'aqua."
18. Plutarch also relates this anecdote in his "Life of Artaxerxes" (chapter 5, 1013 B–C), as did Plutarch's admirer Aelian, who brought out this story in his *Varia Historia* (I.32). But Longo most likely took it from Plutarch's *Moralia,* as the context surrounding the anecdote in that text best fit his own usage and meaning; it was the example Plutarch adduced in urging the emperor Trajan to look kindly on the small but well-meaning gift of his "Sayings of Kings and Commanders" *(Regum et Imperatorum Apothegmata),* which ultimately comprised part of book III of the *Moralia.*
19. Plutarch, *Moralia III, 172B,* trans. Frank Cole Babbit (Cambridge, MA: Harvard University Press, 1961).
20. Arnaldo Momigliano, *Alien Wisdom: The Limits of Hellenization* (Cambridge: Cambridge University Press, 1975), especially chap. 6, "Iranians and Greeks."
21. Margaret Meserve, *Empires of Islam in Renaissance Historical Thought* (Cambridge, MA: Harvard University Press, 2008).
22. Ibid., 218.
23. Niccolò Machiavelli, *The Prince,* ed. and trans. Peter Bonadella (Oxford: Oxford University Press, 2008), especially chaps. 6, 14, and 26.
24. See Lucette Valensi, "The Making of a Political Paradigm: The Ottoman State and Oriental Despotism," in *The Transmission of Culture in Early Modern Europe,* ed. Anthony Grafton and Ann Blair (Philadelphia: University of Pennsylvania Press, 1990), esp. 181 and 187–199. In a similar vein, Achille Olivieri argues that the Ottoman Empire formed a constitutive part of sixteenth-century Venetian political identity; see his *"Esperienza" e "Civiltà" a Venezia nel Cinquecento. L'intelletuale e la città* (Milan: Edizioni Unicopli, 2002), 48–49 and 127–128.

25. On dedications of Plutarch, see Elizabeth McCahill, *Reviving the Eternal City: Rome and the Paper Court, 1420–1447* (Cambridge, MA: Harvard University Press, 2013), 51–55 and 176; see also Elizabeth McCahill, "Finding a Job as a Humanist: The Epistolary Collection of Lapo da Castiglionchio the Younger," *Renaissance Quarterly* 57, no. 4 (2004): 1314–1316. See also Celenza, "Parallel Lives," 121–155; Giustiniani, "Sulle Traduzioni Latine"; Pade, "Sulla Fortuna," 101–116.
26. See especially Israel Abrahams, ed., *Hebrew Ethical Wills* (Philadelphia: Jewish Publication Society, 2006); Mark Cohen, ed. and trans., *The Autobiography of a Seventeenth-Century Rabbi: Leon of Modena's* Life of Judah, 2nd ed. (Princeton, NJ: Princeton University Press, 1989), 48, 55–57, and 174–178.
27. Longo, 1552: "non imprestate ad alcuno sia che esser si voglia, ne danari, ne altro, se p[rim]a non vi pensiate diventarli nemici, per tal imprestido, o non haver mai piu tal cosa a loro prestata, havendone da me esperientia, e pur per non mancar de caritade, fino a ducati cinque a qualechuno piu che amico o parente, (che alcuno de simili si puo ritrovar bisognoso) gli prestarete non piu pensandoli, de tal imprestido, come di cosa non mai facta da voi."
28. Ibid.: "In reliquis vi esorto che nelle cose vostre tutte, cosi grande, come piciole, debbiate dimandar aperto all'omnipotente Dio Sig. Nostro Messer Jesu Christo, che vi favorisca, Essendo a tutti benigni; a niuno lusinghevoli, a pochiss[imi] familiari, molto tarde al'ira, ma prontiss[imi] alla misericordia, et pietade, nelle vostre cose adverse patienti; et nelle prospere continenti; nel far delle ationi vostre prudenti, humili, et accorti."
29. Hadot, *Inner Citadel,* chap. 10 for characteristic practices; quotation at 257.
30. Longo, 1552: "in tutte le sue operatione cosi piccole come grande habbino aparer inanzi li ochi sin il fine di quella operation perche come dice un savio del mondo quella cosa e bona che ha bon fin, et peropposito quella e cativa che ha cativo fin."
31. Ibid.: "mie carissimi et amantissimi fioli quali prego che pensino di non haver heredita alcuna acioche se industriano chi a una [et] chi a un'altra per guandagnarsi el viver et cercar di viver con le sue industrie et virtu."
32. Diomedes Bonardo, ed. and trans., *Galeni Opera* (Venice: Filippo Pinzi, 1490). For mention of Bonardo, and for an excellent overview of Galen's Renaissance translators and emenders, see Stefania Fortuna, "Galenus Latinus, 1490–1533," *Medicina nei secoli* 17, no. 2 (2005): 469–506.
33. Bonardo, *Galeni Opera,* sig. aa1: "ego Diomedes Bonardus phisicus brixiensis omni studio summaque diligentia percurrens Galieni libros . . . sit Platone testante: neque spe lucri deum testor hoc ego peregi: sed tantum doctrine innitens ac veritate: nullam esse existimans neque meliorem hominibus neque divinorem possessionem."
34. Will of Michele di Muti, ASV Notarile Testamenti (Longin), B.1200, n.134: "desiderando esser sepulto piu humil[men]te . . . sia posibile, volendo sop[r]a ogni altra cosa esser posto nel chaileto senza ornamenti de sorte alchuna, eccetto li libri che se sogliano mettere a noi dottori quando semo sepulti, ben

voglio che in reliquis sia osservato come si suole alle sepulture nostre, cioe congregare tutti li Ecc[ellentissi]mi physici de Coleggio nella giesa, et che da uno de detti Ecc[ellentissi]mi physici me sia fatto con la solita mercede la oratione et non da frati volendo sia Ecc[ellentissi]mo Messer Zuane Azian mio char[issim]o comp[ar]e e quello che dovera far la sodetta oratione funerale."

35. Longo, 1574.
36. Nancy Siraisi, *Medieval and Early Renaissance Medicine: An Introduction to Knowledge and Practice* (Chicago: University of Chicago Press, 1990), 20–21.
37. Francesco degli Angeli, ASV Notarile Testamenti (Alchier), B.12, n.93; Vettore Bonagente, ASV Notarile Testamenti (Alchier), B.12, n.222; Alvise Bognolo, ASV Notarile Testamenti (Bianco), B.79, n.15; Antonio Appolonio, ASV Notarile Testamenti (Ziliol), B.1256, n.57.
38. Ottavian Monaldi, ASV Notarile Testamenti (Bianco), B.81, n.837; Andrea Baranzon, ASV Notarile Testamenti (Ziliol), B.1256, n.84.
39. Fiornovella Balsi, ASV Notarile Testamenti (Bianco), B.79, n.405.
40. Franceschina Massa Zuchareda, ASV Notarile Testamenti (Michieli), B.646, n.354.
41. Longo, 1574: "I miei libri, non voglio che si vendano, ma a Pietro mio fiolo lasso tutti li latini, et greco; et gli volgari a Nonio Cornelio, con questa condition, che alcuno de loro, non gli possino alienar, ma tenerli per uso suo, et di suoi posteri et descendenti, et inventariati, possino per l'ultimo herede, o descendente, da essi esser lasciati, a uno monast.o quale habbia libraria per uso de frati, overo altri, overamente alli frati che tenessero Giulio mio fiolo predetto."
42. Household inventory of Pietro Longo (October 17, 1608), ASV Giudici di Petizion, Inventari, B.343, n.93.
43. AAUP, Sacro Collegio dei Filosofi e Medici ("Tomo Estraordinario"), n.403, fols.1–4. Hereafter AAUP.
44. Ibid., testimony of Acharius Stat, f.1r: "erat aromatarius insigne pomi de aurati, et ibi stabat t[a]nq[quam] factor, deinde tanq[uam] patronus fuit una[m] appoth[ecam] aromatariae ad insigne testis aurati sup[er] Campo S[an]ti B[a]rth[olom]ei."
45. Ibid., testimony of Pelegrino, fol.1v: "multi anni erat aromatarius in Apotheca ad insigne Pomi Deaurati, et erat Ille . . . gubernator in dicta apotheca / Deinde fecit unam appoth[ecam] aromat[ar]i[a]e ad insigne Capitis Aurati."
46. Ibid., testimony of Pietro, fol.3r: "era spiciale a la insegna de la testa doro."
47. An excellent example of the use of this phrase appears in the fifteenth-century physician-humanist Giovanni Caldiera's discussion of "magnificence," discussed by King, *Venetian Humanism,* 100–101.
48. AAUP, testimony of Pelegrino, fol.1v: "era uno homo da bene, et fecce gran facende" and testimony of Pietro, fol.3r: "era uno homo da bene, et fecce gran facende a dicta sua botega de spiciarie."
49. Lauro Martines, *The Social World of the Florentine Humanists, 1390–1460* (Toronto: University of Toronto Press, 2011), esp. 6–12, 31, 198, 261–262, and 329.

50. AAUP, testimony of Alessandro Rugerio, fol.2r: "fr[atris] dicti D. Franc[esch]i Longi fuit ele[va]tus ad ipsum Cancellarium."
51. Longo, 1574: "Al ditto monasterio lasso tutto quello che paresse debitore per li libri de mio fratello, et miei, per conto de medicine havute alla sua spiciaria, fino alla morte del ditto mio fratello."
52. Will of Bernardin Ramboso (August 16, 1556), ASV, Notarile Testamenti (Atti Bianco), B.78, n.181.
53. An excellent recent analysis of social mobility in Renaissance Florence is John F. Padgett, "Open Elite? Social Mobility, Marriage and Family in Florence, 1282–1494," *Renaissance Quarterly* 63, no. 2 (Summer 2010): 357–411.
54. See especially Jonathan Dewald, *The European Nobility, 1400–1800* (Cambridge: Cambridge University Press, 1996), 33–36; and Matthew Lundin, *Paper Memory: A Sixteenth-Century Townsman Writes His World* (Cambridge, MA: Harvard University Press, 2012), 125ff.
55. An excellent critical edition of this text is Poggio Bracciolini, *De vera nobilitate,* ed. Davide Canfora (Rome: Edizioni di Storia e Letteratura, 2002). For a recent approach ongoing literary debates concerning nobility, see Claudio Finzi, "La polemica sulla nobiltà nell'Italia del Quattrocento," *Cuadernos de Filologîa Clásica. Estudios Latinos* 30, no. 2 (2010): 341–380.
56. On the famous botanical garden and its contemporary impact, see Margherita Azzi Visentini, *L'orto botanico di Padova e il giardino del Rinascimento* (Milan: Polifilo, 1984).
57. BNM, "Notizie tratte dai Libri dei Priori," MS It. VII, 2342 (=9695), fol.6v: "1531 . . . Primo luglio, ingresso di Francesco Longo senza bal[l]ottaz[ione]." Hereafter BNM, "Notizie." Before midcentury, it was not that unusual for new members to enter the College without a formal vote (after 1550, by contrast, this was very rare). Indeed, this same year two other physicians joined the College without balloting: Raphael da Cortona and Francesco Butiron (ibid.). Joining the College without any formal voting, however, does suggest that the candidate already had strong supporters among the established members.
58. For Longo's terms as treasurer, see the account book of Benedetto Rini, in which we find receipts of Rini's annual college dues recorded in the hand of each year's new treasurer, IRE, "Quadernetto di varie ricevute 1513–1552," DER E, B.189, fasc.6 (unfoliated), entries dated July 3, 1534, and April 21, 1543. For Longo's priorates, BNM, "Notizie," fols.80v and 81r.
59. In 1514, for instance, the College denied a young doctor the salary reserved for "experts," despite the fact that Venice's captain general Andrea Gritti had chosen him as personal physician. BNM, "Notizie," fol.2r: "1514, p[rim]o giugno. Contesa tra il Prior e il Cap[itano] Gen[erale] Andrea Griti che avea eletto per suo medico un troppo giovine et inesperto, perciò il col[legi]o non voleva darli il salario, che si dava agli esperti."
60. On sexual slander among intellectuals, see Lauro Martines, *Strong Words: Writing and Social Strain in Renaissance Italy* (Baltimore, MD: Johns Hopkins

University Press, 2001); Ingrid Rowland, "Revenge of the Regensburg Humanists, 1493," *Sixteenth Century Journal* 25, no. 2 (Summer 1994): 307–322; Elizabeth McCahill, "Humanism in the Theater of Lies: Classical Scholarship in the Early Quattrocento Curia" (PhD diss., Princeton University, 2005), 105–112 and 158–192. On attacks in the "Republic of Letters" more generally, see Anthony Grafton, *Worlds Made by Words: Scholarship and Community in the Modern West* (Cambridge, MA: Harvard University Press, 2009), 14–16 and 34.

61. AAUP, fol.2r.
62. Ibid., fol.4r: "Fidem facio Ego presbiter Joannes Renius iu[ris] ut[rumque] doc[toris] Ecclesi[a]e S. Jacobj de Luprio Venet. qualiter D[ominu]s Petrus d[e] Longis qu[ondam] D[omi]ni Girardj est venetus & natus est in S. Jacobj et Luprio ut publice habemus & [regarding his sons' legitimacy] de quo tamen nihil habemus in s[cri]ptis."
63. Ibid., fol.1r: "Et primo interrogatus se cognovit patrem dicti D. Franc[esc]i Longi, et cuius nomen erat, i[u]r[amen]to suo respondit . . . possu[n]t esse anni Triginta sex . . . cognovit patrem dicti D. Franc[esc]i nomine Petrum, et erat ipsius testis Comparer . . . Dixit elevasse a sacro fonte p[re]fatum D[ominum] Franc[escu]m sive eius fratrem, quia non bene meminir an testis ipse elevaverit dict[um] D[ominum] Franc[escu]m an fratrem eius, Dicens 'forse che io li ho levadi tuti dui che ben non me ricordo.'"
64. Celenza, "What Counted as Philosophy?"
65. Longo, 1574: "Impero ordinar voglio di esse ancorche poche el desiderio mio, accio dapoi la mia morte non habbino cagione li posteri et heredi miei di litigar tra loro, ma viver pacificamente. Quali sopra tutte le altre cose esorto, et prego ad haver tra essi la pace lasicata dal Sig. nostro messer Jesu Christo a soi discepoli, et a tutti noi, con la quale se contentaranno di quello che Io haverò ordinato, et faranno come amorevoli fratelli, et miei figlioli carissimi."
66. On superfluous sons, see especially Stanley Chojnacki, *Women and Men in Renaissance Venice: Twelve Essays on Patrician Society* (Baltimore, MD: Johns Hopkins University Press, 2000), 244–256.
67. Will of Marietta Longo (1566), ASV, Notarile Testamenti (Bianco), B.80, n.742: "tuttj vadino in Piero Julio et Cornclio mie fiolj."
68. Palmer, *Studio of Venice,* 145.
69. Longo, 1574: "non nomino Giulio in tal offitio, ancor che sia mio figliolo, come li sopradetti [Pietro and Cornelio] per non esser idoneo a tal cosa per natura"; "non voglio che Giulio se habbi ad imp[egn]ar di governo alcuno per non esser atto a questo, come è notissimo."
70. Ibid.: "con questa condizione, che a Giulio vostro fratello faciate le spesse, vestendolo et calciandolo, come si dice et governandolo insieme da frattello con voi, si insieme habiarete, se non in casa di quello di voi, che lui vorà, havendone de lui quel governo che si richiede a frattelli, et questo facio, accio non essendo esso Giulio ad alcuna cosa atto, ne ancora a governar se medesmo, come è a molti notiss.o. Possi lui vivere con quel honor, che potrà insieme con voi, la qual cosa vi comando, protesto et per le [visc]ere di messer Jesu Christo

vi prego lo faciate; pensandovi, che se Dio havesse permesso, peggio molto, et voi, et tutti noi potressimo esser di quel che è lui, della natura creati, come de molte altre chiaramente si vede."

71. Ibid., sig.G6v: "Sola autem natura eos humores, quibus mediis agglutinantur, & postea simul coalescunt vulneratae partes, tanquam aptam, & congruentem materiam potest subministrare: medicus vero, aut nihil aut parum. Praeterea vero & concretio & coalitus ille, non nisi opera naturae fit, & caloris nativi, qui aut ipsamet natura est, aut eius proximum instrumentum. Medicus tamen tanquam eius adiutor, & minister illam in hoc opere potest iuvare." Other physicians, as well as the commonality, in Europe and elsewhere even construed medicine as a gift from God. See Paul F. Ramírez, "Minerva's Mexico: Science, Religion and the Art of Healing in Late Colonial Epidemics, 1736–1850" (PhD diss., University of California, Berkeley, 2010).
72. Longo, 1574: "eccetuato però Giulio mio fiolo predetto per non esser capace, ne di ordine, ne di ragione, et potria con lieve persuasioni esser ingannato a maleficio suo, et de altri."
73. See Guido Ruggiero, *Binding Passions: Tales of Magic, Marriage and Power at the End of the Renaissance* (New York: Oxford University Press, 1993); Erik Midelfort, *Witchcraft, Madness, Society and Religion in Early Modern Germany: A Ship of Fools* (Aldershot, UK: Ashgate Variorum, 2013).
74. Jonathan Seitz, *Witchcraft and Inquisition in Early Modern Venice* (Cambridge: Cambridge University Press, 2011), 149–168.
75. Longo, 1574: "Quando veramente esso Giulio volesse andar, come spesse volte ha detto, in monasterio, in quel caso, inteso bene el voler suo, et ottimamente [pensata] tal casa et da lui, et da voi, vi consiglio a riponerlo, dando alli frati dove lo mettesti quella elimosina, che vi paresse, con cautela però, come si conviene quale mi penso saperete fare, accio per tal cosa havessero causa li frati de tenerlo, e fagli bona compagnia, et lui di starvi volontieri."
76. Longo, 1552: "Alli mie carissimi fioli lasso in aricordo et precetto tre cose."
77. Michel Foucault, *Madness and Civilization: A History of Insanity in the Age of Reason,* 2nd ed. (New York: Routledge, 2001).
78. Elizabeth Mellyn, *Mad Tuscans and Their Families: A History of Mental Disorder in Early Modern Italy* (Philadelphia: University of Pennsylvania Press, 2014). See also David Gentilcore, *Healers and Healing in Early Modern Italy* (Manchester: Manchester University Press, 1998); Mary Lindemann, *Medicine and Society in Early Modern Europe* (Cambridge: Cambridge University Press, 1999).
79. On married women's "dissociation" from their natal families, see Christiane Klapisch-Zuber, *Women, Family and Ritual in Renaissance Italy,* trans. Lydia G. Cochrane (Chicago: University of Chicago Press, 1987), esp. 117–131 and 213–246; Margaret King, *Women of the Renaissance* (Chicago: University of Chicago Press, 1991), 61–62.
80. Elissa Weaver, *Convent Theater in Early Modern Italy: Spiritual Fun and Learning for Women* (Cambridge: Cambridge University Press, 2002); K. J. P. Lowe, *Nuns' Chronicles and Convent Culture in Renaissance and Counter-Reformation Italy*

(Cambridge: Cambridge University Press, 2003); Dava Sobel, *Galileo's Daughter: A Historical Memoir of Science, Faith and Love* (New York: Bloomsburg Publishing, 1999); Mary Laven, *Virgins of Venice: Broken Vows and Cloistered Lives in the Renaissance Convent* (New York: Penguin, 2004), 93 and 116; Sharon Strocchia, *Nuns and Nunneries in Renaissance Florence* (Baltimore, MD: Johns Hopkins University Press, 2009), 39–71, 167–176, and 186–188.

81. Daniel Bornstein, ed. and trans., *Life and Death in a Venetian Convent: The Chronicle and Necrology of Corpus Domini* (Chicago: University of Chicago Press, 2000), 5 and 16–17.
82. Laven, *Virgins of Venice,* 50.
83. On the Vergini, see Lowe, *Nuns' Chronicles,* 299–317. See also Laven, *Virgins of Venice,* 78–79.
84. ASV, Corpus Domini: (Carta/Paper) B.2, "Instrumento de Livello . . . Priuli" (1604—Longo is eighth of forty-two nuns, not counting the prioress); B.4, fasc.28 (1605—sixteenth of twenty-four nuns); (Pergamene/Parchment), B.5, fasc.1 (1562—Longo is thirty-ninth of forty nuns); B.5, fasc.3 (1593—Longo is twelfth of thirty-eight nuns); B.6, "Valier" (1601—Longo is eleventh of forty nuns); B.6, "Basadonna" (1603—Longo is ninth of fifty-two nuns); B.6, "Solari" (1603—Longo is ninth of fifty-one nuns); B.6, "Finasola" (1607—Longo is eighth of forty-three nuns).
85. ASV, Corpus Domini, B.26 (Carta), tab in account book "Venuto e Speso 1668–1704," under which we see periodic payments of twenty-five lire to a "M[adre] Spitiera."
86. Sobel, *Galileo's Daughter,* 9, 112–119, 209–210, and 325.
87. Bornstein, *Life and Death,* 16 and 27; quotation at 27.
88. Laven, *Virgins of Venice,* 50–51.
89. Ibid., 26–27; Paul Grendler, *The Roman Inquisition and the Venetian Press, 1540–1605* (Princeton, NJ: Princeton University Press, 1977), 18.
90. On the social effects of sixteenth-century and early seventeenth-century dowry inflation, see especially Virginia Cox, "The Single Self: Feminist Thought and the Marriage Market in Early Modern Venice," *Renaissance Quarterly* 48, no. 3 (Autumn 1995): 513–581; Jutta Sperling, *Convents and the Body Politic in Late Renaissance Venice* (Baltimore, MD: Johns Hopkins University Press, 1999).
91. Household inventory of Orfeo Copazzo (1584), ASV, Giudici di Petizion, Inventari, B.338, n.42.
92. Longo, 1552.
93. ASV, Corpus Domini (Pergamene), B.5, item marked "Instrumento di M. Marchio dei Schuteri," dated July 7, 1562.
94. Longo, 1574: "Ordino et cosi voglio, che a mia fiola Suor Virginia, monaca nel monasterio del Corpus Domini per li miei commissarij predetti, gli sia dato ogn'anno fino che viverà . . . ducati cinque . . . Voglio ancora che a madonna Suor Theodosia monaca in ditto monasterio sia dato ogni anno fino che viverà ducati uno . . . ancor che poco et quasi niente sia a quello che meriterà, per l'amorevolezza che porta a mia fiola, ma questo faccio per signal

d'aricordo, et non per ricompensa de meriti." Suor Theodosia was most likely Theodosia Bottoni, who appears in the roll call of nuns assembled to chapter in October 1557: ASP, Monalium, Documenti Diversi 1-9, 1377-1795, fasc.4 "Corpus Domini"; document dated October 31, 1557.

95. Longo, 1574: "prima per l'amorevolezza, et bontade de esse monache, la seconda accio che mia fiola monaca in detto monastero sia da esse governata amorevolmente, come fin hora è stata."
96. Ibid.
97. Longo, 1552.
98. Ibid.
99. Pietro Longo did follow his father into the medical profession, even without prodding. BNM, "Elenco Priori e Dottorati," Ms. It. VII, 2379 (=9686), fol.18v.
100. Basegio di Lazari, ASV Notarile Testamenti (Bonifacio Solian), B.937, n.174: "Per mei chomesarii . . . volgio che sia messer Franzescho di Longi de le arte et medizina dotor mio nepote."
101. Will of Marietta Longo, ASV, Notarile Testamenti (Bianco), B.80, n.742: "io Marieta consorte del Ecc[ellent]e phisico Messer Francesco Longo."
102. ASV, Corpus Domini, B.5, fasc.16, "San Marcilian: Piero Longo per la q[onda]m Suor Virginia. Consumate, Cassella no.12": "Con[stitu]ito nell'offitio Domino Oratio Longo in sua specialita et come commesario della comessaria del quondam M[ess]er Basilio di Lazari." The household inventory for Pietro Longo also provides a detailed survey of his papers, which indicate that he had been married once and, after the death of his wife, had contracted a second marriage, but there are no indications of blood heirs.
103. Inventory of Pietro Longo's household goods and papers, ASV, Giudici di Petizion, Inventari, B.343/8, n.93: "quali tutte robbe si ritrovo haver indosso [Pietro Longo] nella casa del sud[ett]o messer Pietro di Schietti, com[messa]rio dove passo a miglior vita supradetto S[igno]r[e] Pietro fatte portar nella casa della sua habitacion."
104. ASV, Proveditori sopra la sanità, B.809, entry under the parish heading (San Marcilian) dated August 31, 1576: "L'Eccellente Messer Francesco di Longo fisico da febri in nota li 26."
105. Household inventory of Pietro Longo, ASV, Giudici di Petizion, Inventari, B.343/8, n.93: "Una testa de piera cota disie esser l'effigii del qu[ondam] S[ignore] Francesco Longo."
106. Longo stipulated that his funeral and burial should be as economical as possible, with total expenses kept under forty ducats (Longo, 1574).

5. CULTURAL LIFE IN THE JOURNALS OF ALBERTO RINI

1. For excellent synthetic treatments of the intellectual history of medicine, see especially A. Wear, R. K. French, and I. M. Lonie, *The Medical Renaissance of the*

Sixteenth Century (Cambridge: Cambridge University Press, 2009); Nancy Siraisi, *Medieval and Early Renaissance Medicine: An Introduction to Knowledge and Practice* (Chicago: University of Chicago Press, 1990); and Nancy Siraisi, *History, Medicine and the Traditions of Renaissance Learning* (Ann Arbor: University of Michigan Press, 2007).

2. Bryon Grigsby, *Pestilence in Medieval and Early Modern English Literature* (New York: Routledge, 2004); Louise M. Bishop, *Words, Stones, Herbs: The Healing Word in Medieval and Early Modern England* (Syracuse, NY: Syracuse University Press, 2007).
3. Gianna Pomata, *Contracting a Cure: Patients, Healers and the Law in Early Modern Bologna* (Baltimore, MD: Johns Hopkins University Press, 1998).
4. Elizabeth Cohen, "Miscarriages of Apothecary Justice: Un-Separate Spaces for Work and Family in Early Modern Rome," and Felippo de Vivo, "Pharmacies as Centres of Communication in Early Modern Venice," in *Spaces, Objects and Identities in Early Modern Italian Medicine,* ed. Sandra Cavallo and David Gentilcore (Oxford: Wiley Blackwell, 2008), 8–32 and 33–49, respectively; Patrick Wallis, "Consumption, Retailing and Medicine in Early Modern London," *Economic History Review* 61, no. 1 (2008): 26–53. For a new approach to "trading zones," see Pamela Long, *Artisan/Practitioners and the Rise of the New Sciences, 1400–1600* (Corvallis: Oregon State University Press, 2011).
5. See especially Nancy Siraisi, *Communities of Learned Experience* (Baltimore, MD: Johns Hopkins University Press, 2012).
6. Alberto Rini, "Giornali," ASV, Scuola Grande di San Marco, B.112, fasc. 1. Again, I express my thanks to Beth and Jonathan Glixson for bringing this source to my attention.
7. For the rise of "free literates," see Armando Petrucci, *Writers and Readers in Medieval Italy: Studies in the History of Written Culture,* ed. and trans. Charles M. Radding (New Haven, CT: Yale University Press, 1995), 173–179.
8. James Grubb, "Memory and Identity: Why Venetians Didn't Keep *Ricordanze,*" *Renaissance Studies* 8, no. 4 (1994): 375–387.
9. Matthew Lundin, *Paper Memory: A Sixteenth-Century Townsman Writes His World* (Cambridge, MA: Harvard University Press, 2012).
10. Ibid., 25–26 and 97–98. On the problem of bachelorhood, see also Stanley Chojnacki, *Women and Men in Renaissance Venice: Twelve Essays on Patrician Society* (Baltimore, MD: Johns Hopkins University Press, 2000), 244–256.
11. Alberto Rini, Giornali, ASV Notarile Testamenti, Scuola Grande di San Marco, B.112, fasc.1, Giornale A (unfoliated), entry dated August 12, 1559: "Isabella mia figliola morise et stete inferma giorni 13." Hereafter, I will refer to the two account books as "Giornale A" and "Giornale B."
12. Giornale B, fol.28v: "Per un breviario Romano quasi nuovo comprato a R[ial]to per mandar a mia figliuolin a Sibinico, 16 soldi."
13. Ibid., fol.36r: "Per una casselletta depenta di verde da mandar a Seb[eni]co a mia figlioccia, 2 lire."
14. Ibid., f.155r: "Il Ser.mo P. DD Pasqual Cigogna ad hore 16 in circa passo' di questa vita, havendo vissusto nel Dogado Anni 9 M7 D15, et il Martedi si pub.

io' la sua morte, et il Venere furono celebrate le pompe funerali in chiesa di SSti Gio: et Paolo, et l'oratione funebre fù fatta dall'Ecc.te M. Enea Piccolho[min]i denese, Lettor pub.co qui in Ven.a et il cadavero fù portato a sepellire alli Crocieri."

15. Giornale A, entry dated August 3, 1560: "El Nostro Can satin morise alhora 19 et e stato sepelito in corte in la altavola dal Jesmin appresso el lauro Marina fece l'offitio."
16. Benedetto Rini testament (1563), IRE, DER E, B.189, fasc.1, n.14: "Alberto nella sua terza parte habbia ducati correnti Dusento et cinquanta de più de gli altri, da esser tolti cento et cinquanta della parte di Fabricio, et cento della parte de Scipion, et questo per haver speso in quelli in mantenerli in studio in Padoa, et dottorarli et quelli cinquanta da esser cavadi della parte di Fabritio lui sa molto ben, perche voglio, che lui habbia consummado della sua parte terza. Appresso voglio, che quello mio libro depento de Simplici sia sempre d'Alberto, et questo per bon respetto, pregando Alberto non lo vogli privar di casa, ne fidarsi di darlo fuori delle sue mani, per esser una cosa rara." On the precious herbal, see also Francesca Pitacco, "Un prestito Mai Rifuso: La vicenda del *Liber de simplicibus* di Benedetto Rini," in *Fibure di collezionisti a Venezia tra Cinque e Seicento* (Udine: Forum, 2002), 11–23.
17. Giornale B, fol. 91v: "Nel giorno dell'Epifania ad un hora di giorni in ca. nascettero dui figlioli maschi in uno partato alla Cl.ma Sra. Elisabetta Miani, moglie del Cl.mo Sr. Zacc.a Valaresso fu del Cl.mo messer Alvise qu' è nostro vicino, et alli 12 del detto mese furono ambidue figliuolini battezati in chiesa di S. Provolo per mano del Rdo. messer P. Giac.o Sasso nostro capellano et li furno compari in nro. di 22 fra tutti dui, fra' quali li tenge M. Scipione mio fratello."
18. Ibid., fol.118v.
19. Ibid., fol. 98v: "Faccio memoria, come in questo giorno M. Scipione mio fratello fù ballottato nella Scuola di messer S. Marco, per commiss.o del q. messer Piero Vinier, et rimase con ballotte no.18 et otto di nò, et io era uno delli xviij et fù in concorso di messer Bartolomeo Moro Avocato, messer Marco Zon, messer Hieronimo di Francesci et di messer Andrea Dardani, in qual commissaria tra' da dar via 24 case à Sta. Maria Maggior, insieme con due altri commissarij, li quali sono al presente messer Cesare Ziliol, et messer Marc'Antonio Gerardo."
20. Ibid., fol. 113v: "Mro. Marc'Antonio de Bortolo Calafado di Venetia fù messo questo anno in Scuola di S. Marco, con il mezo del Cl.mo sr. Franc.o Gerardo Sec.o del C. di X. et fù messo gratis, et amore per causa nostra."
21. Ibid., fol.86v: "Faccio nota, come con il mezzo del Cl.mo Sr. Fco. Gerardo Segretario dell'Ecc.te Consiglio di X.i feci metter in Scuola di S. Marco senza premio alcuno un mio figliuoccio nominato Tomaso calafado."
22. Ibid., fol.144r–v: "14 January 1593 [4]. Noto, come in questo giorno, che fù di Venere si maritò la Mag.ca Mad.a Bortolamia da Ca' di Piero mia nezza, fi-

gliola che fù del S. Hier.o mio cugino, et tolse per marito il S. Gadi Gadi gentilhuomo di Forlì, il qual starà qui in Venetia et è mercati ricchissimo, et stà alla Maddalena in Ca' Molino. prego nostro S. Iddio, che le dia felicita et buona ventura. [. . .] 25 January 1593[4]. Con il nome di Dio, Padre, figliolo et spirito Sancto si diede la mano alla Mag.ca Madonna Bertolamia figliola che fù di messer Gier.o da Ca' de Piero mio cugino, et lei viene ad essere mia nezza, la qual si maritò nel Sr. Gadi Gadi da Forlì con dote di 6M ducati, et piu, et andò la medesima sera a casa del novizzo, la quale era in Monasterio di S. Hier.o a spese et ciò ho notato per memoria. Lo sposo stà in Ca' Molino alla Maddalenna."

23. Ibid., fol.151r.
24. Ibid., fol.149v: "Queste sono le parole che sono nella capella appresso la sagrestia a Crocecchieri delli test.i da Seda, dove vi sono ritratti [. . .] delli Sri. di quell'Arte, et fra quali vi si trova M. Alberto da Rin mio Avo come dalle inscrittione si lege cioè: Giacomo de Simone, Antonio de Varisco, Filippo de Beltramo, Giacomo de Bortolamio, Zuanne de Georgi, Alberto da Rin, Fermo de Stefano, Nicolò de Marco, Michiel Vezo, Alessio. Lattantio da Rimino D. 1. B. P. 1499."
25. Ibid., fol.187r.
26. Lundin, *Paper Memory,* 182–185.
27. The literature on the gift is vast, but some particularly useful studies with wide scope are the following: Marcel Mauss, *The Gift: Forms and Functions of Exchange in Archaic Societies,* trans. Ian Cunnison (London: Taylor and Francis, 2002); Natalie Zemon Davis, *The Gift in Sixteenth-Century France* (Oxford: Oxford University Press, 2000); Jane Lawson, *The Elizabethan New Year's Gift* (Oxford: Oxford University Press, 2013); for Italy more particularly and for learned exchange, see Christiane Klapisch-Zuber, *Women, Family and Ritual in Renaissance Italy* (Chicago: University of Chicago Press, 1985), esp. 213–246; J. Cunnally, "Ancient Coins as Gifts and Tokens of Friendship during the Renaissance," *Journal of the History of Collections* 6, no. 2 (1994): 129–143.
28. Giornale B, fol.71v.
29. Giornale A (end).
30. Giornale B, fol.46v.
31. BNM, "Notizie tratte dai Libri dei Priori," MS It. VII, 2342 (=9695), f.81v.
32. BNM, MS It. VII, 2342 (=9695), fol.15r.
33. Vettore Trincavella, *Opera omnia* (Lyons: Giunti and Paolo Guitti, 1586), sig.+5r. See also Apostolo Zeno's transcription of Marucini's Vita of Trincavella in Zeno's collection of notes on famous Venetians, BNM, MS It. VII, 351 (=8385), fol.456v.
34. Trincavella, *Opera omnia,* vol. 1 (unsigilated preface).
35. Alvise Luisin, ed., *De morbo gallico, omnia quae extant apud omnes medicos cuiuscunque nationis,* 2 vols. (Venice: Giordano Ziletti, 1566–1567), vol. 2, sigs.Bb1v et seq.

36. For Fabrizio Rini's dedication, see ibid., vol. 2, sig.Bb1v.
37. Record of Rini's funeral (May 1566) appears in BNM, "Notizie Tratte dai Libri dei Priori," MS It. VII, 2342 (=9695), fol.14r: "Esequie di Benedetto Rin alli Frati Minori. Fece l'oraz. Alvise Luisin. furono quasi tutti li Medici."
38. Trincavella, *Opera omnia,* sig. *2v: "An ego illum defunctum, & in medio templo iacentem siccis oculis intueri unquam possem? an sine gravi gemitu tam pij mihi praeceptoris funus comitari deberem? Qui me filij loco semper habuit, cuius moribus & doctrina vel a' puero institutus."
39. Diana Robin, *Publishing Women: Salons, the Presses and the Counter-Reformation in Sixteenth-Century Italy* (Chicago: University of Chicago Press, 2006).
40. On the changing conceptions of copying and note taking, see Ann Blair, *Too Much to Know: Managing Scholarly Information before the Modern Age* (New Haven, CT: Yale University Press, 2010), 108–112. For an early typology of writerly endeavor that was already making value distinctions between "mere" copying and creative writing, see also Petrucci, *Writers and Readers,* esp. 149.
41. Giornale A (unfoliated), miscellaneous notes made in conclusion to the journal, which ends in 1574.
42. Giornale B, fols.49r–51v.
43. Ibid.
44. Dandolo's chronicles appear in Ester Pastorello, ed., *Chronica per extensum descripta,* in *Rerum italicarum scriptores,* 2nd ed. (Bologna: Zanichelli, 1939). For analysis of the chronicles in the wider context of early-modern historical writing, see Sharon Dale, Alison Williams Lewin, and Duane J. Ostreim, eds., *Chronicling History: Chronicles and Histories in Medieval and Renaissance Italy* (University Park: Pennsylvania State University Press, 2009), esp. 200–204. On Dandolo's broader cultural contributions, see Debra Pincus, "Hard Times and Ducal Radiance: Andrea Dandolo and the Construction of the Ruler in Fourteenth-Century Venice," in *Venice Reconsidered: The History and Civilization of an Italian City State, 1297–1797,* ed. John Martin and Denis Romano (Baltimore, MD: Johns Hopkins University Press, 2000), 89–136; Patricia Fortini Brown, *Venice and Antiquity: The Venetian Sense of the Past* (New Haven, CT: Yale University Press, 1996), 34–43; Henry Maguire and Robert S. Nelson, *San Marco, Byzantium and the Myths of Venice* (Cambridge, MA: Harvard University Press, 2010), esp. 246. See also the seminal article of Lino Lazzrini, "'Dux ille Danduleus': Andrea Dandolo e la cultura veneziana a metà del Trecento," in *Petrarca, Venezia e il Veneto, Civiltà veneziana, Saggi 21,* ed. G. Padoan (Florence: Olschki, 1976), 123–156.
45. Giornale B, fol.93r.
46. On the centrality of history to very different intellectual currents, see especially Anthony Grafton, *What Was History? The Art of History in Early Modern Europe* (Cambridge: Cambridge University Press, 2007), chap. 3; see also Siraisi, *History, Medicine and the Traditions.*
47. Rini inventory (1604), IRE, DER E 189, fasc.3, n.30.

48. For Maxson's definitions, see *The Humanist World of Renaissance Florence* (Cambridge: Cambridge University Press, 2014), 10–11; for importance of correspondence networks, see esp. 79–81; on humanism as a form of social ritual, see 92–106 and 133.
49. On Ramusio and Mercuriale, see Siraisi, *History, Medicine and the Traditions,* 49.
50. Will of Scipione Rini, ASV, Notarile Testamenti (Atti Secco), B.1192, n.566.
51. Giornale B, fol.101v (January 9, 1588–1589): "Per un libro de gli Imp[erator]i Nerva, Traiano et Adriano, et altri tradotti de Gio: Battista Egnatio comprato a Rialto di Stampo d'Aldi."
52. Ibid., fol.93v: "Havi, con il mezo del Mag[nifi]co S[igno]r[e] Paolo Ramusio un'officietto della Madonna mandatomi di Francia dal S[igno]r[e] Gier[olem]o suo figliuolo, che era secret[ari]o a quella M[aes]tà Cristianissima con il Cl[arissi]mo S[igno]r[e]. Zuanne Dolfino, et è di stampa di Anversa del 1586, coperto di cuoro rovano con un filetto d'oro attorno."
53. Ibid., fols.67r–68v.
54. Blair, *Too Much to Know,* 114–115.
55. Giornale B, "per quinterni di carta da scrivere le prediche," entries begin May 20, 1592, and appear at intervals of every few months thereafter, fols. 132r, 133v, 138v, 140r, 144r, 146r, 150v, and 153r.
56. Ibid., fol.144r: "Ho dato al Mag.co S. Nicolò Caroldo 20 quinternetti delle prediche del Rdo. Brisighella, da mandare al Rdo. D. Giacomo di Conti monaco a S. Michiel in Padova."
57. Long, *Artisan/Practitioners;* Pamela Long, *Openness, Secrecy, Authorship: Technical Arts and the Culture of Knowledge from Antiquity to the Renaissance* (Baltimore, MD: Johns Hopkins University Press, 2004), esp. chap. 5; William Eamon, *Science and the Secrets of Nature: Books of Secrets in Medieval and Early Modern Culture* (Princeton, NJ: Princeton University Press, 1996); William Eamon, *The Professor of Secrets: Mystery, Medicine and Alchemy in Renaissance Italy* (Des Moines, IA: National Geographic Books, 2010).
58. For the materiality of writing and, as part of that, the problem of inks and mounts (from the twelfth century onward), see Bernhard Bischoff, *Latin Palaeography: Antiquity and the Middle Ages* (Cambridge: Cambridge University Press, 1990), esp. 16–18.
59. Giornale B, for paper and ink purchases, see, for instance, fols. 50r, 85r, 133v, 140r, 143r, 147v, and 150v; for Rini splashing out on the higher-quality ink, see fol.143r.
60. Ibid., f.69r: "Recetta da far inchiostro negrissimo et ottimo havuta dal S[igno]r[e] Dom[eni]co Salis / Piglia Gomma Arabica onze una / Vitriolo Romano onze due / Galla d'Istria onze tre / Vino bianco tondo ottimo onze 33/ Bisogna dar una rotta sol[amen]te alla galla, et poi metter il tutto insieme a boglire per due soli bogli, et sarà fatto, et riuscirà perfettissimo."
61. Deborah Harkness, *The Jewel House: Elizabethan London and the Scientific Revolution* (New Haven, CT: Yale University Press, 2007).

62. Giornale B, fol.79r: "Agliata da fare in tempo di peste usata dal Sr. Abbate di Sacco lungo. Pigliate pn. dal basilico, dell'herba buona, et tagliate il tutto minuto, et poi bisogna pigliar uno spico d'aglio cotto sotto le ceneri, et pestar il tutto insieme, tolendo poi due, o tre molene di pane bagnato nell'acqua, et mettendogli delle noci, et poi pestate il tutto benissimo et poi stemperate ogni cosa con l'agrestà et così è fatta, triandola un poco, et tutto deve esser freddo. Et alcuni metteno dell'aceto in cambio d'agresta, et è rara et effettissima." In a similar vein, Rini had gleaned a cure for kidney stones, which he attributed to "the Reverend pres of San Giorgio Maggiore"—see ibid., fol.81r.
63. Ibid., fol.12r and insert.
64. Ibid., fols. 81r, 95r, and 132r, respectively.
65. Ibid., fol.115r.
66. Ibid., f.11v (August 8, 1576): "per dar al medico della contrada L3s2."
67. Patrick Wallis, "Plagues, Healers, and Patients in Early Modern Europe," *Renaissance Quarterly* 52, no. 2 (1999): 474–486.
68. In particular, Rini's journals note payments of rent to him roughly every six months from the "Reverend pres of Sant'Elena" in the amount of thirteen ducats and eighteen soldi (Giornale B, inter alia fols. 128v and 170r. The rental agreement with the priest of Sant'Elena seems to have been formed in 1591, as the payments commence then.)
69. See especially Mary Lindemann, *Medicine and Society in Early Modern Europe* (Cambridge: Cambridge University Press, 1999), 193–230.
70. Giornale B, fol.16v.
71. Ibid., fol.35v. On guiac, see Siraisi, *History, Medicine and the Traditions,* 173–174; Lindemann, *Medicine and Society,* 57; Jon Arrizabalaga, John Henderson, and Roger French, *The Great Pox: The French Disease in Renaissance Europe* (New Haven, CT: Yale University Press, 1997), 100–104 and 230–255.
72. Giornale B, fol.44r–v.
73. Ibid., fol.49v.
74. Ibid., fol.180v.
75. Ibid., fol.84r, entry dated December 1586.
76. Ibid., fol.127v.
77. Giornale A, entries dated June 7, 1563, and February 15, 1563–1564.
78. Giornale B, fol.10r: "Noto, come in questo giorno fù serrato il monasterio di S[an] Zacharia per causa di una monaca, che morì et fu lei data di sospetto dalli Medici, et questo io noto per memoria, che nostro Signor Dio per sua Divina misericordia non permetti tal flagello procedere più oltre."
79. On "deformazione professionale" see Lisa Jardine and Anthony Grafton, "'Studied for Action': How Gabriel Harvey Read His Livy," *Past and present* 129 (1990): 30–78; for a contrasting view, see Douglas Biow, *Doctors, Ambassadors, Secretaries: Humanism and the Professions in Renaissance Italy* (Chicago: University of Chicago Press, 2002), esp. x–xii.
80. Giornale B, fol.51r: "Messer Hier[olem]o di Piero nostro cugino passò di questa vita, essendo stato ammalato da dui anni in circa di male Ettico."

81. Giornale A, entry dated December 9, 1565: "Morise il santissimo Papa nostro Pio iiii de casa Medici in giorno di Domenica ad hore quatro di notte et morì di mal colico."
82. Giornale B, fol.119v: "IHS MARIA / Adi 14 novembre 1590/ Noto faccio io Alberto come sotto di ditto il mio carissimo et dolcissimo fratello messer Scipion passò di questa all'altra vita che nostro Sr. Dio habbi misericordia all'anima sua. Et la sua infirmità fù di un'accidente gagliardissimo di Apolessia che in termine di hore nuove, terminò la sua vita, et si cominciò l'accidente la mattina ad' hora di mezza terza et all'Ave Maria della sera chiuso gli occhi in un sempiterno sonno."
83. Nicolò Massa, *De febre pestilentiali* (Venice: Andrea Arrivabene, 1555), sig. C4v (for his father's death) and C5r for his brother's: "tale genus febris passus est doctissimus et carissimus frater meus Thomas Massa, qui in quarta defecit cum omnibus accidentibus fortibus, & apostemate inguinis, q. cognovi licet eo tempore nondum essem medicus."
84. For writing as retreat, see Pierre Hadot, *The Inner Citadel: The* Meditations *of Marcus Aurelius* (Cambridge, MA: Harvard University Press, 2001), 265.
85. Will of Scipione Rini, IRE, DER E, B.189, fasc.1, n.36.
86. Giornale A, poem appears (twice) in a cluster of notes in the final folios.
87. Jason Saunders, *Justus Lipsius: The Philosophy of Renaissance Stoicism* (New York: Liberal Arts Press, 1955); Jill Kraye, "The Revival of Hellenistic Philosophies," in *The Cambridge Companion to Renaissance Philosophy*, ed. James Hankins (Cambridge: Cambridge University Press, 2007), 97–112; Arnaldo Momigliano, "The First Political Commentary on Tacitus," *Journal of Roman Studies* 37 (1947): 91–101, esp. 98; for the development of the "Senecan style," see 100. For a more recent approach, see Christopher Brooke, *Philosophic Pride: Stoicism and Political Thought from Lipsius to Rousseau* (Princeton, NJ: Princeton University Press, 2012). See also Mark Morford, *Stoics and NeoStoics: Rubens and the Circle of Lipsius* (Princeton, NJ: Princeton University Press, 1991).
88. Hadot, *Inner Citadel,* esp. 48–51, 257–259, and 313.
89. Giornale B, fol.20v: "Si suonò campanna à martello dalle 20 sino alle 3 di notte in campanile di S. Mco. et il giorno per tutte le contrate di Vinetia. Furono subbito deputati molti Nobili et Cittadini armati alla guardia delle strade, che vengono in piazza si nel gorno, come nella notte. furono anco accesi infiniti torzi et lumiere per la piazza et candele di cera erano accese sopra tutti li balconi delle case nuove et vecchie. Mai nel ricordo d'huomo è stato il maggior, et il più horendo incendio di questo, et durò sino alle sette di notte."
90. Ibid.: "per le orationi del Beatissimo Vangelista et Prottettor nostro messer S. Marco, fece, che il vento abbonacciò, et così la chiesa et il resto rimase intatto. il fuoco cominciava a penetrare all'Off.o del Procur.o et Mobele, ma per virtù et industria, certo, rara, della Maestranza, non puote far progresso."
91. Ibid.: "tutte le due sale grandi si brusiarono, et insieme insieme le pitture eccl. me et del Bellino et dell'Titiano et il soffito, con frattura delli due pergoli et di cascare molte colonne delli balconi che erano di belleza rare."

92. Ibid., fol.104r.
93. Ibid., fol.31r.
94. Ibid., fol.72r: "Fù tagliata la testa tra le due colonne a S. Gabriel Emo . . . qual era [?] della Sforzade, havendo tagliato à pezzi molti Turchi, et alcune donne di sangue Regio d'Algier, et toltole la robba, li danari, et le gioie, et la [sententia] fù fatta dall'Ecc.mo Cons.o di preg.i la sera avanti."
95. Ibid., fol.75v: "Noto, come li Giapponesi Indiani sono entrati nella Scuola della Carità, et li furono donati da S. Grande 4 candelotti miniati, et la sua cuppa fornita, il qual dono fu loro gratissimo et hanno detto di voler eriggere nel suo paese una fraterna simile."
96. Judith Brown, "Courtiers and Christians: The First Japanese Emissaries to Europe," *Renaissance Quarterly* 47, no. 4 (1994): 872–906.
97. Ibid., 905. For discussion of Venetian perspectives, see 900–901.
98. On Venetian political pageantry, see Edward Muir, *Civic Ritual in Renaissance Venice* (Baltimore, MD: Johns Hopkins University Press, 1986).
99. Giornale A, entry dated March 11, 1570 (1571 in modern reckoning): "Fu fatto Dose de Venetia messer Alvise Mocenigo . . . et fu portato el sabbado da mattina per piazza trazando delli denari in pergoletto segondo l'usanza antica, et era lui vestito di panno d'oro come cavallier, et haveva in comp[agni]a doi soi fratelli, nevodi fioli de doi soi fratelli, et è stato benissimo visto da tutto el populo et si tiene per fermo, che lui sarà un gloriosissimo Dose, et forse non minor del q. Ser.mo Gritti de felice memoria per 3 giorni continoi si sono in S. Marco et si fece che molti fughi per la città, et el ditto è maridato in una da ca Marcello, et così si haverà Dogaressa."
100. Giornale B, fol.17r.
101. Ibid.: "Fù eletto [. . .] il Cl.mo messer Sebastian Venier [. . .] di S. Moisè et è da notar che li 41 entrarno in conclave la mattina del marti, et il dopò disnar elessero Dose il sopradetto messer Sebastian Venier, che fù del 1571 Nostro Capitano qual da mar nel giorno della solennissima et memorabilissima Vittoria havuta contra Turchi, et hebbe tutti li voti delli 41 cosa che mai più si ha inteso, il che fù con estrema allegrezza di tutta la città."
102. Ibid., fol.22r: "Il Ser.mo Principe DD Sebastian Venier Morì, il qual stette in dogado solamente mesi otto et giorni 20 et è stato ammalato se non giorni otto di una crisipela nella testa, Et era di anni 82 et fu con dolor la sua morte a tutta la città et fù sepulto honorevolissimamente a Sta. Maria di Anz.li da Muron."
103. Ibid.: "era una piogga incredibile, dove furono astretti a fare le dette esseq[i]e a S. Marco."
104. Giornale A, entry dated April 5, 1570: "fu odiado da tutto il populo de Venetia dicendo che lui è stato c[aus]a della carestia, mortalità, guerra et incendio dell'Arsenale, et fu sepulto nella chiesa de S. Iseppo."
105. Hadot, *Inner Citadel,* 257–300.
106. For the claim that Marcus wrote only for himself, see ibid., 34 and 50; for a slightly different conceptions of Marcus's intended audience as an abstract

"transcendent Other," see 121–122; and for the third notion of the audience as Marcus's higher self, see 301.

107. Duccio Balestracci, *The Renaissance in the Fields: Family Memoirs of a Fifteenth-Century Tuscan Peasant,* trans. Paolo Squatriti and Betsy Merideth (University Park: Pennsylvania State University Press, 1999), xix.
108. Petrucci, *Writers and Readers,* 189.
109. Lundin, *Paper Memory,* 36, 162–163, and 205.

CONCLUSION

1. David Herlihy, "Three Patterns of Social Mobility in Medieval Society," *Journal of Interdisciplinary History* 3 (1973): 623–647; quotation at 646.
2. John Padgett, "Open Elite? Social Mobility, Marriage and Family in Florence, 1282–1494," *Renaissance Quarterly* 63, no. 2 (2010): 357–411, esp. 380.
3. Ibid., 402.
4. Dennis Romano, *Patricians and Popolani: The Social Foundations of the Venetian Renaissance State* (Baltimore, MD: Johns Hopkins University Press, 1987), esp. 50–54.
5. Alexander Cowan, *Marriage, Manners and Mobility in Early Modern Venice* (Aldershot, UK: Ashgate Publishing, 2007), esp. 67–90.
6. For the claim that a humanistic education had an "ornamental" value for men and women, as the disjunctures between literary accomplishments and their possessors' daily activities and types of employment often made this style of education primarily valuable "for its own sake," see Anthony Grafton and Lisa Jardine, *From Humanism to the Humanities: Education and the Liberal Arts in Fifteenth- and Sixteenth-Century Europe* (Cambridge, MA: Harvard University Press, 1986), 43–44 and 57.
7. Peranda will, ASV Notarile Testamenti, B.1259, n.563: "Lasso a Zuanbattista . . . studiando come spero tutti li miei libri et ogni altra cosa appartenente al mio studio."
8. There were no standard legal protocols for adopting children in Renaissance Italy. Men and women might take in orphans when the deceased parents happened to be their kin, friends, or neighbors. We also sometimes see cases of men and women taking in children from foundling homes, though this was rare compared with the number of cases in which unwanted or orphaned offspring were deposited in such institutions. See especially Nicholas Terpstra, *Abandoned Children of the Italian Renaissance: Orphan Care in Florence and Bologna* (Baltimore, MD: Johns Hopkins University Press, 2005).
9. Ibid. See also Foscarini will: "alli quali quanto io posso raccomando il sopradetto Zuanbattista facendolo sopra il tutto studiar, acciò [che] el deventa Ecc.te, et homo da bene, et honorato."
10. Francesca Zan Benetti, ed., *Acta graduum academicorum gymnasii Patavini ab anno 1601 ad annum 1605, Fonti per la storia dell'Università di Padova* (Padua:

Editrice Antenore, 1987), 5:177. He may also have followed his adoptive father in an openness to or even adherence to heterodox beliefs. Richard Palmer has noted that Giovanni Battista Peranda (the elder) had to flee Venice to avoid an Inquisitional trial. See Richard Palmer, "Physicians and the Inquisition in Sixteenth-Century Venice: The Case of Girolamo Donzellini," in *Medicine and the Reformation,* ed. Ole Peter Grell and Andrew Cunningham (London: Routledge, 1993), 119. Peranda (the younger) had as one of his *promotores* Cesare Cremonini, repeatedly denounced to the Inquisition, whose works were also on the Index of Prohibited Books. See Jonathan Seitz, *Witchcraft and the Inquisition in Early Modern Venice* (Cambridge: Cambridge University Press, 2011), 185–186.

11. Seitz, *Inquisition,* 155, 160, and 186n50.
12. A fine English rendering of this letter appears in Francesco Petrarch, *Letters on Old Age (Rerum senilium libri)*, trans. Aldo S. Bernardo, Saul Levin, and Reta A. Bernardo (New York: Italica Press, 2005), 1:672–680.
13. For a splendid analysis of this letter and, more broadly, Cicero's conception of posterity as an act of writing, see Andrew Lintott, *Cicero as Evidence: A Historian's Companion* (Oxford: Oxford University Press, 2011), 215–424.
14. Matthew Lundin, *Paper Memory: A Sixteenth-Century Townsman Writes His World* (Cambridge, MA: Harvard University Press, 2012), 33–49, 163–164, and 226–228.
15. On conceptions of audience in family documents, see ibid., 226–227.
16. William Sherman, *Used Books: Marking Readers in Renaissance England* (Philadelphia: University of Pennsylvania Press, 2007).
17. Jeffrey Todd Knight, *Bound to Read: Compilations, Collections and the Making of Renaissance Literature* (Philadelphia: University of Pennsylvania Press, 2013).
18. Dana Sajdi, *The Barber of Damascus: Nouveau Literacy in the Eighteenth-Century Ottoman Levant* (Stanford, CA: Stanford University Press, 2013), esp. chap. 2.
19. Paula Findlen, "Ereditare un museo. Collezionismo, strategie familiari e pratiche culturali nell'Italia del XVI secolo," *Quaderni Storici* 115 (2004): 45–81; see also Marino Zorzi, "La circolazione del libro a Venezia nel Cinquecento: biblioteche private e pubbliche," *Ateneo veneto* 177 (1990): esp. 137–139.
20. Isabella Palumbo Fossati, *L'interno della casa dell'artigiano e dell'artista nella Venezia del Cinquecento* (Pisa: Giardini Editori e Stampatori, 1984), 131; discussed in Zorzi, "Circolazione," 129.
21. On prints, see especially Isabella Cecchini, "Collezionismo e mondo materiale," *Il collezionismo d'arte a Venezia* 2 (2008): 165–191; Michael Bury, *The Print in Italy, 1550–1620* (London: British Museum, 2001).

ACKNOWLEDGMENTS

While I cannot speak for "man," I do know that no researcher is an island. Accordingly, first thanks go to my colleagues at Boston College, and especially to the outstanding cadre of premodernists, intellectual historians, and Europeanists there, scholar-teachers who model excellence in their own research and have been exceedingly generous with their time in engaging mine. My heartiest thanks go to Julian Bourg, Mary Crane, Robin Fleming, Sylvia Sellers-García, Kevin Kenny, Stephanie Leone, Prasannan Parthasarathi, Devin Pendas, Owen Stanwood, Dana Sajdi, Philipp Stelzel (now of Duquesne University), and above all Virginia Reinburg, whose positive influence appears on every page.

I am also beholden to many scholars outside the BC biosphere—Kenneth Gouwens, Anthony Grafton, Paula Findlen, Laurie Nussdorfer, William Monter, Elizabeth McCahill, Edward Muir, and Diana Robin—for reading and critiquing early drafts. In this same category of exemplary readers, however, my deepest thanks go to Kate Lowe for her astute guidance in reshaping the exposition at a critical moment in its life as a manuscript and, after she assumed the editorship of the I Tatti Studies in Italian Renaissance History series at Harvard University Press, for championing the project as a potential contribution to that series.

Speaking of the Press, I thank the two anonymous readers, whose enthusiasm and insightful critiques gave me just the right blend of encouragement and direction for undertaking the final revisions. Thanks as well to Andrew Kinney and Katrina Vassallo at Harvard University Press for guiding the project to and through production, and to the team at Westchester Publishing Services for their swift and careful copyediting.

Scholarly books need considerable research support even before their first sentences get typed, let alone published. I would therefore like to express my gratitude to the Gladys Krieble Delmas Foundation for enabling me to spend 2010–2011 in the Venetian archives, as well as to the department and university administrators at Boston College for permitting me to shirk my usual teaching and departmental responsibilities that year.

Upon arriving in the Veneto, I gleefully capitalized on the expertise of staff at many repositories, but Dott. Francesco Piovan of the Archivio Antico della Università (Padova) and Dott.ssa Agata Brusegan of the Archivio IRE (Venezia) went far beyond the call of duty to connect me with archival treasures. And I heap blessings on Beth and Jonathan Glixson, fellow habitués of the Archivio di Stato di Venezia, for alerting me to the *giornali* of Alberto Rini. What these scholars found to be "not terribly useful" for their own studies proved, as they suspected, revelatory for mine. Also in Venice, for many invigorating conversations and for introducing me to her family, I thank Marina del Negro Karem.

In the realm of my own kin, huge thanks go to my parents, Robert and Sandra Ross. Librarians by training and voracious readers, my parents harbor an interest in book people, and of course in their fledgling. All the same, their unflagging support and the many hours spent listening to material from or tales about this project, as well as their many excellent suggestions, must be classified as altruism. Broadening the definition of *kinship* a bit, I would like to acknowledge several friends who ensure that I continue to nurture other interests. By sharing the ballet studio with me, or luring me out of my fetid lair with new ideas, works of literature, performances, and other adventures, Ginny Reinburg, Louise Grafton, Arthur Leeth, Sejal Patel, and Andrea Schatz have in their various ways saved me from becoming entirely Gollum-like.

In the end, however, perhaps those who most need acknowledgment are this study's protagonists, whose hopes for inclusion in the sort of world that I too often take for granted have by turns inspired and chastened me. I am especially grateful to His Excellency Francesco Longo, physician and philosopher, for dictating the enigmatic wills that started this adventure. I hope this book may in some measure repay my debt to him, and to all the aspiring humanists I have had the honor of meeting, whether on the page or in person. *Grazie di cuore.*

INDEX